T0320458

Cloud Computing Systems and Applications in Healthcare

Chintan M. Bhatt
Charotar University of Science & Technology, India

S. K. Peddoju
Indian Institute of Technology Roorkee, India

A volume in the Advances in Healthcare Information Systems and Administration (AHISA) Book Series

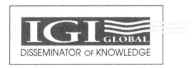

www.igi-global.com

Published in the United States of America by
    IGI Global
    Medical Information Science Reference (an imprint of IGI Global)
    701 E. Chocolate Avenue
    Hershey PA 17033
    Tel: 717-533-8845
    Fax: 717-533-8661
    E-mail: cust@igi-global.com
    Web site: http://www.igi-global.com

                    Library of Congress Cataloging-in-Publication Data

Names: Chintan, Bhatt, 1988- editor. | Peddoju, S. K., 1973- editor.
Title: Cloud computing systems and applications in healthcare / Chintan Bhatt
    and S.K. Peddoju, editors.
Description: Hershey, PA : Medical Information Science Reference, [2017] |
    Includes bibliographical references and index.
Identifiers: LCCN 2016028110| ISBN 9781522510024 (hardcover) | ISBN
    9781522510031 (ebook)
Subjects: LCSH: Medicine--Data processing. | Cloud computing. | Mobile
    computing.
Classification: LCC R858 .M623 2017 | DDC 610.285--dc23 LC record available at https://lccn.loc.
gov/2016028110

This book is published in the IGI Global book series Advances in Healthcare Information Systems and Administration (AHISA) (ISSN: 2328-1243; eISSN: 2328-126X)

British Cataloguing in Publication Data
A Cataloguing in Publication record for this book is available from the British Library.

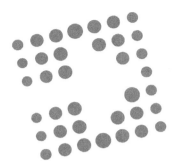

Advances in Healthcare Information Systems and Administration (AHISA) Book Series

ISSN: 2328-1243
EISSN: 2328-126X

MISSION

The **Advances in Healthcare Information Systems and Administration (AHISA) Book Series** aims to provide a channel for international researchers to progress the field of study on technology and its implications on healthcare and health information systems. With the growing focus on healthcare and the importance of enhancing this industry to tend to the expanding population, the book series seeks to accelerate the awareness of technological advancements of health information systems and expand awareness and implementation.

Driven by advancing technologies and their clinical applications, the emerging field of health information systems and informatics is still searching for coherent directing frameworks to advance health care and clinical practices and research. Conducting research in these areas is both promising and challenging due to a host of factors, including rapidly evolving technologies and their application complexity. At the same time, organizational issues, including technology adoption, diffusion and acceptance as well as cost benefits and cost effectiveness of advancing health information systems and informatics applications as innovative forms of investment in healthcare are gaining attention as well. **AHISA** addresses these concepts and critical issues.

COVERAGE

- Decision Support Systems
- Management of Emerging Health Care Technologies
- Rehabilitative Technologies
- IT Applications in Physical Therapeutic Treatments
- Virtual Health Technologies
- IT Security and Privacy Issues
- Telemedicine
- Pharmaceutical and Home Healthcare Informatics
- Role of Informatics Specialists
- IS in Healthcare

IGI Global is currently accepting manuscripts for publication within this series. To submit a proposal for a volume in this series, please contact our Acquisition Editors at Acquisitions@igi-global.com or visit: http://www.igi-global.com/publish/.

Titles in this Series

For a list of additional titles in this series, please visit: www.igi-global.com

Reshaping Medical Practice and Care with Health Information Systems
Ashish Dwivedi (University of Hull, UK)
Medical Information Science Reference • copyright 2016 • 399pp • H/C (ISBN: 9781466698703) • US $150.00 (our price)

M-Health Innovations for Patient-Centered Care
Anastasius Moumtzoglou (P&A Kyriakou Children's Hospital, Greece)
Medical Information Science Reference • copyright 2016 • 438pp • H/C (ISBN: 9781466698611) • US $235.00 (our price)

Improving Health Management through Clinical Decision Support Systems
Jane D. Moon (The University of Melbourne, Australia) and Mary P. Galea (The University of Melbourne, Australia)
Medical Information Science Reference • copyright 2016 • 425pp • H/C (ISBN: 9781466694323) • US $225.00 (our price)

Maximizing Healthcare Delivery and Management through Technology Integration
Tiko Iyamu (Cape Peninsula University of Technology, South Africa) and Arthur Tatnall (Victoria University, Australia)
Medical Information Science Reference • copyright 2016 • 378pp • H/C (ISBN: 9781466694460) • US $235.00 (our price)

Flipping Health Care through Retail Clinics and Convenient Care Models
Amer Kaissi (Trinity University, USA)
Medical Information Science Reference • copyright 2015 • 306pp • H/C (ISBN: 9781466663558) • US $245.00 (our price)

Healthcare Informatics and Analytics Emerging Issues and Trends
Madjid Tavana (La Salle University, USA) Amir Hossein Ghapanchi (Griffith University, Australia) and Amir Talaei-Khoei (University of Technology, Sydney, Australia)
Medical Information Science Reference • copyright 2015 • 414pp • H/C (ISBN: 9781466663169) • US $235.00 (our price)

Laboratory Management Information Systems Current Requirements and Future Perspectives
Anastasius Moumtzoglou (Hellenic Society for Quality and Safety in Healthcare, Greece & P. & A. Kyriakou Children's Hospital, Greece) Anastasia Kastania (Athens University of Economics and Business, Greece) and Stavros Archondakis (Military Hospital of Athens, Greece)
Medical Information Science Reference • copyright 2015 • 354pp • H/C (ISBN: 9781466663206) • US $245.00 (our price)

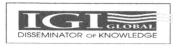

www.igi-global.com
701 E. Chocolate Ave., Hershey, PA 17033
Order online at www.igi-global.com or call 717-533-8845 x100
To place a standing order for titles released in this series,
contact: cust@igi-global.com
Mon-Fri 8:00 am - 5:00 pm (est) or fax 24 hours a day 717-533-8661

Editorial Advisory Board

Table of Contents

Detailed Table of Contents

Chapter 1
Veda Prakash Mangu, Graphene Semiconductors Ltd., India

This chapter gives a high-level view of the technology involved in the solution of Mobile Health Care with Cloud Computing as back-bone. It emphasizes on Hardware elements, Computation requirements when the solution covers huge scope of medical problems at the mega scales across wide areas. This chapter discusses subsystems of the solution, that include Smart Phones, Computation Engines, High End Transportation Systems, Multi-Specialty Hospitals, Smart Phones/Digital Personal Assistants used by Medical Practitioners. Discusses on the accuracies, bandwidth requirements and latencies present in the systems, also emphasizes on the required accuracies as the problem area is Human Life. To address the challenges that arises when the solution gets high degree of maturity, this chapter proposes review of the current day protocols in the systems. Also proposes to integrate intelligent applications and different eco-systems like Big Data, Data Analytics and Internet of Things, and best adaptability of these areas with Nano-technologies to result in increased average life time of humans.

    Ajay Chaudhary, Indian Institute of Technology Roorkee, India
    Sateesh Kumar Peddoju, Indian Institute of Technology Roorkee, India
    Suresh Kumar Peddoju, Kakatiya Institute of Technology and Science,
        India

The wireless infrastructure based devices can collect data for long period of time even with a tiny power source as they perform specific function of collection of health related data and sending to gateways. The sensing data of healthcare monitoring consumes low power but they had limited computation power to process this data, where the cloud computing plays a vital role and compliment the loophole of wireless infrastructure based systems. In cloud computing with its immense computation power for easily deployment of healthcare monitoring algorithms and helps to process sensed data. As these two technologies did great jobs in their respective fields a conflate framework of these two technologies may lead to a great architecture for healthcare applications. This chapter reviews complete state-of-the-art and several use cases related to healthcare monitoring using different wireless infrastructure and adapting cloud based technologies in providing the healthcare services.

    Saravana Kumar N., VIT University, India
    Rajya Lakshmi Gubburi Venkataramana, Northwestern Polytechnic
        University, USA
    Balamurugan B., VIT University, India

Cloud computing is one of most fast developing technology and many organizations are now offering a wide range of cloud services. Although the services provided are the same there is no common programming language, technology and protocol to access the entirety of the cloud services. Client who use a service provided by a certain organization are often limited and confined to that specific organization its structure and technologies. A Cloud federation is one solution to that interoperability through which computing resources of one Cloud Service Provider is rented or sold to another service provider or the services provided by one Cloud Service Provider is replicated into another Cloud Service Provider without having to lose any functionality and performance. This process is a tedious task and is prone to multiple limitations. In this paper we proposed the architectural framework and algorithm for the possible interoperability between the cloud service providers based on SLA in prospective of health sector as the application of cloud in health sector is highly needed in future.

Chapter 4

Drashti Dave, Central University of Rajasthan, India
Nagaraju Aitha, Central University of Rajasthan, India

In the current Information Technology virtualization is one of the key components during the performance evaluation of network enabled environment including distributed computing, cloud computing, grid computing or pervasive computing. The network administrators and forensic teams are working on software defined networking (SDN) using which the network components can be controlled and managed using virtual infrastructure and global view of the physical network. On the physical implementation viewpoint, the single error or oversight can be damage the entire network integration. Now days, the advent of SDN products are being used in the research, development and corporate industry so that the effective control including routing, scheduling, security and related algorithms can be implemented on real networks. There are number of real life applications where the software defined networking and service oriented architecture (SOA) can be implemented for the social and global cause. Medical and Health Care Service is one of the key domain can make use SDN approach in which the number of medical decisions are to be taken based availability of the enterprise information. In this research work, the case analysis and a prototype for health care management service is accomplished. In this chapter, a unique and pragmatic implementation of the SDN based on virtualization is done and the prototype which we proposed in this chapter will be validated in future by using mininet-openflow integration to evaluate the performance of network and data packets transmission.

Chapter 5

Suresh Kumar Peddoju, Kakatiya Institute of Technology and Science, India
Kavitha K., Indian Institute of Technology, India
Sharma S. C., Indian Institute of Technology, India

In developing countries pediatric pneumonia is the second leading cause of deaths and 98% of pneumonia-induced deaths are identified across the world. It is mandatory to identify the symptoms of pneumonia in children to avoid mortality causing complications. Early identification of children at risk for treatment failure or at increased risk for death will help to improve overall health outcomes. If pneumonia is suspected, it is important to seek medical attention promptly so that an accurate diagnosis can be made and appropriate treatment is given in time. The proposed approach quickly provides history of previous patient's details, expert doctor's opinions who are in globe and their previous treatment for the same symptoms, all diagnostic reports such as blood tests, x-ray etc., from the cloud and gives analytics from big data to take fast and precise decisions by the doctors.

Chapter 6

The healthcare system is important due to the focus on human care and the interference with human lives. In recent years, we have witnessed a rapid rise in e-healthcare technologies such as Electronic Health Records (EHR) and the importance of emergency detection and response. Cloud computing is one of the new approaches in distributed systems that can handle some of the challenges of smart healthcare in terms of security, sharing, integration and management. In this study, an architecture design of a cloud-based pervasive healthcare system for diabetes treatment has been proposed. For this, three different components are defined as follows: (1) The home context manager which gathers necessary information from patients while simultaneously providing feedback, (2) a patient health record manager that is accessible by nurses or physicians at the hospital, and (3) a diabetes management system which is located with the cloud infra-structure for managing and accessing patient's information. The performance of proposed architecture is demonstrated through a user scenario.

Chapter 7

With the advent of Internet and Computers, Information Technology (IT) has become a major tool to aid medical issues. IBM Watson is one such initiative by IBM, which provides integration with any application to build Internet of Things (IoT), based health applications and also assists by its existing services. The strength of Watson is its data analytics and Artificial Intelligence. The four variants of Watsons are Watson Discovery Advisor, Oncology, Clinical Trial Matching and Curam. It is based on Open Source Apache UIMA, Apache Lucene. Its integration with IBM Bluemix Cloud, Platform as a Service (PaaS) makes it easily available to users.

Chapter 8

Cloud Computing changes the way data innovation (IT) is expended and oversaw, promising enhanced cost efficiencies, quickened advancement, quicker time-to-market, and the capacity to scale applications of interest. Users have started to explore new ways to interact with each other with the omnipresent nature of Social Networks and Cloud Computing. Facebook, YouTube, Orkut, Twitter, Flickr, Google+, Four Square, Pinterest, and the likes have distorted the way the Internet (Social Cloud) is being used. However, there is an absence of comprehension of protection and security issues of online networking. The protection and security of online networking should be explored, concentrated on and portrayed from different viewpoints (PCs, social, mental and so on). It is basic to distinguish security dangers and shield protection through constant and adaptable frameworks. Subsequent to there is no intelligent limits of the social networking, it is vital to consider the issue from a worldwide viewpoint as well.

In recent era individuals and organizations are migrating towards the cloud computing services to store and retrieve the data or services. However, they have less confidence on cloud as all the task are handled by the service provider without any involvement of the data owner. Cloud system provides features to the owner, to store their data on some remote locations and allow only authorized users to access the data according to the role, access capability or attribute they possess. Storing the personal health records on cloud server (third party) is a promising model for healthcare services to exchange information with the help of cloud provider. In this chapter, we highlight the various security issues and concerns such as trust, privacy and access control in cloud based healthcare system that needs to be known while storing the patient's information over a cloud system.

Health care institution demands exchange of medical images of number of patients to sought opinions from different experts. In order to reduce storage and for secure transmission of the medical images, Crypto-Watermarking techniques are adopted. The system is considered to be combinations of encryption technique with watermarking or steganography means adopted for safe transfer of medical images along with embedding of optional medical information. The Digital Watermarking is the process of embedding data to multimedia content. This can be done in spatial as well as frequency domain of the cover image to be transmitted. The robustness against attacks is ensured while embedding the encrypted data into transform domain, the encrypted data can be any secret key for the content recovery or patient record or the image itself. This chapter presents basic aspects of crypto-watermarking technique, as an application. It gives a detailed assessment on different approaches of crypto-watermarking for secure transmission of medical images and elaborates a case study on it.

In the modern fast and stressful life, an individual does not have time to take an extra care for one's self. Support from general information about health and nutrient requirement through modern computing infrastructure is very limited and common. Generic information on the Web and other media sometime raises genuine queries about the good health. Further, typical solutions available may not interact with users in friendly way and deal with vague inputs provided by users. To resolve this issue, a system is required which knows its users, acts smartly and friendly, learns from past data & history and provides customised advisory. This chapter introduces a neuro-fuzzy architecture, based on which an expert system for determination of nutrient requirements is presented. The chapter includes in depth literature survey, concepts, implementation details with sample code, neural network structure, fuzzy membership functions used, sample input–output screens of the system and future work.

Foreword

LinkedIn is networking without the pressure of having to wear a name tag, meet strangers and awkwardly attempt a small talk for introduction, writes Ms. Melaine Pinalo. This is exactly how I was connected to Prof. Chintan Bhatt. Holding similar research interests, it is my pleasure to introduce his new work titled "Cloud Computing Systems and Applications in Healthcare". The book comes to publishing in the interesting digital era of intelligent computing & data driven information architecture where current health care decision makers around the globe are looking for guidance regarding evaluating cloud computing offerings. In the past from working with pharmacy companies in cloud migration projects, I personally have observed the key acceleration factor for cloud adoption in health care industry is widely influenced by achievements the early adopters showcase and claim. On those chords, I believe the book has interesting case studies and lessons learnt to offer from the practitioner's perspective.

Prof. Chintan Bhatt is an academician with numerous publication to add to his accolades. He has chaired and hosted conferences related to cloud computing, knowledge engineering and internet of things. His wisdom and approach has influenced well in pulling such related case studies into a book. Dr. Sateesh is a famous academician in the areas of cloud computing, mobile systems, computer networking and operating systems. He has served as editor, expert committee member and as part of board of studies.

On demand access of cloud is a popular enterprising model for compute resources in an effective new paradigm that helps organizations achieve operational efficiency in a lucrative business context. This book discusses such computational requirements from a medical solution perspective by elaborating on storage, infrastructural, sensor, integration and architectural needs. The book discusses aspects of service level agreements and specific management service dashboards as demanded by healthcare. Specific treatment based case studies regarding how cloud computing offerings were utilized in diabetic cure, cancer cure and medical imaging would be of interest for practitioners looking forward to build new prototypes and systems targeting specific illness or medical domains.

Managing integrated storage when it comes to electronic patient record is becoming the new norm for the healthcare industry. The book provided insights regarding new ways of information processing that is possible from these collected patient health records discussing possibilities of scalable sharing platforms. Innovative analytics based on the preserved big data that will help medical diagnostics are highlighted. Also information security and data privacy aspects that are to be excised during such cloud adoption are being elaborated in details. Secured transmission protocols such as crypto watermarking are being discussed in the context of medical data transmission. A neuro-fuzzy architecture for determining nutrient requirements is also presented and analyzed for benefits.

I wish them best for their book written in pursuit of capturing contextual knowledge of applying cloud computing solutions in healthcare industry.

Suriya Priya Asaithambi
National University of Singapore, Singapore

Preface

INTRODUCTION

Cloud computing has turned into an extraordinary answer for giving an adaptable, on-interest, furthermore, progressively versatile figuring foundation for some applications. Cloud figuring likewise shows a critical innovation patterns, and it is as of now self-evident that it is reshaping data innovation forms and the IT commercial center. The extent of the book incorporates driving edge cloud computing innovations, frameworks, and designs; cloud computing administrations; and an assortment of distributed computing applications.

With the sensational development of cloud computing advances, stages and administrations, this altered can be the conclusive asset for persons working in this field as analysts, researchers, developers, architects, and clients. The book is proposed for a wide assortment of individuals including academicians, originators, designers, instructors, engineers, professionals, analysts, and graduate understudies. This book can additionally be advantageous for business chiefs, business visionaries, and financial specialists. We are appreciative to IGI Global for accepting our book proposition. From that point on it was test to amass thoughts from numerous specialists from different parts of the world into one single book.

This book means to give the most recent exploration discoveries in the territory of virtualization of libraries. The sections of this book are brought about by specialists in this field and clients of this innovation. The creators have utilized their experience to present data which will be a valuable advantage for our objective perusers and experts who are keen on enhancing their comprehension here and who are slanted towards utilizing this innovation as a part of their library to give cloud-based data administrations to their supporters. The book can have an incredible potential to be embraced as a reading material in present and new courses on Cloud computing.

SPECIAL FEATURES

What makes this book special is the solidarity in differing qualities. It is a gathering of musings and thoughts by not one but rather a few creators from different strolls of life. Consequently it incorporates specialists, analysts, IT educationists, IT experts, Cloud experts, all framing an insightful rainbow of learning. The International Review and Editorial group has invested an extraordinary push to build up a quality item for the apprentices and specialists in the Cloud. This book concentrates on the most recent advancement of data innovation and utilization of the Internet, which is 'Cloud Computing' and its application. A person perusing through the book not just acclimates himself with the idea of cloud computing, additionally gets a knowledge on how cloud computing is significant to the society.

STRUCTURE OF THE BOOK

The book is outfitted with enormous data. It contains contextual investigations, models and engineering of applications and improves the perusers with significant data, setting them up to confront their particular expert fields with eagerness to execute the most recent innovation bridled to advantage the curious human personality. The book moreover gives something worth mulling over to pundits around there, empowering them to mull over the issues, concerns and confinements which should be handled with awesome consideration so as to upgrade the advantages of cloud computing in this excited universe of developments and innovative progressions.

Chapter 1 gives a high-level view of the technology involved in the solution of Mobile Health Care with Cloud Computing as back-bone. It emphasizes on Hardware elements, Computation requirements when the solution covers huge scope of medical problems at the mega scales across wide areas.

Chapter 2 reviews complete state-of-the-art and several use cases related to healthcare monitoring using different wireless infrastructure and adapting cloud based technologies in providing the healthcare services.

Chapter 3 proposed the architectural framework and algorithm for the possible interoperability between the cloud service providers based on SLA in prospective of health sector as the application of cloud in health sector is highly needed in future.

Especially nowadays, the advent of SDN products are being used in the research, development and corporate industry so that the effective control including routing, scheduling, security and related algorithms can be implemented on real networks. Medical and Health Care Service is one of the key domain can make use of SDN approach in which the number of medical decisions are to be taken based on availability of the enterprise information. In Chapter 4, the case analysis and a prototype for health care management service is accomplished.

Chapter 5, proposed approach that quickly provides history of previous patient's details, expert doctor's opinions who are in globe and their previous treatment for the same symptoms, all diagnostic reports such as blood tests, x-ray etc., from the cloud and gives analytics from big data to take fast and precise decisions by the doctors.

Chapter 6 provides an architecture design of a cloud-based pervasive healthcare system for diabetes treatment has been proposed. For this, three different components are defined as follows: (1) The home context manager which gathers necessary information from patients while simultaneously providing feedback, (2) a patient health record manager that is accessible by nurses or physicians at the hospital, and (3) a diabetes management system which is located with the cloud infra-structure for managing and accessing patient's information.

Chapter 7 describes how Watson can be used for treating Patients. Watson is an IBM cloud which is used worldwide for treating patients even for diseases like cancer, it has a wide data base and uses features of open source softwares. The chapter covers the details of Watson from very basics to how you can use it.

Chapter 8 introduces the protection and security of online networking. It should be explored, concentrated on and portrayed from different viewpoints (PCs, social, mental and so on). It is basic to distinguish security dangers and shield protection through constant and adaptable frameworks.

Chapter 9 has highlighted the various security issues and concerns such as trust, privacy and access control in cloud based a healthcare system that needs to be known while storing the patient information over a cloud system.

Chapter 10 presents basic aspects of crypto-watermarking technique, as an application. It gives a detailed assessment on different approaches of crypto-watermarking for secure transmission of medical images and elaborates a case study on it.

Chapter 11 introduces a neuro-fuzzy architecture, based on which an expert system for determination of nutrient requirements is presented. The chapter includes in depth literature survey, concepts, implementation details with sample code, neural network structure, fuzzy membership functions used, sample input–output screens of the system and future work.

Chintan M. Bhatt
Charotar University of Science & Technology, India

S. K. Peddoju
Indian Institute of Technology Roorkee, India

Acknowledgment

The editors acknowledge the support and efforts of a number of colleagues. First and foremost, we would like to thank the contributors to this book, the authors and co-authors from academia as well as industry from around the world who collectively developed and submitted chapters. Without their efforts in developing quality chapters conforming to the required guidelines, and meeting often the strict deadlines, this text would not have been possible.

Secondly, our grateful thanks are to the members of the editorial board and reviewers of this book who willingly volunteered their time in reviewing the book chapters and providing further advisory and editorial support.

Finally, we would like to thank our HoD(s)-Computer Engineering Department and colleagues of Indian Institute of Technology, Roorkee and Charotar University of Science And Technology. We would like to thank Jan and IGI Global Team for their continuous support in this project.

Thank you all, most heartily.

Chintan M. Bhatt
Charotar University of Science & Technology, India

S. K. Peddoju
Indian Institute of Technology Roorkee, India

Chapter 1
Mobile Health Care:
A Technology View

Veda Prakash Mangu
Graphene Semiconductors Ltd., India

ABSTRACT

This chapter gives a high-level view of the technology involved in the solution of Mobile Health Care with Cloud Computing as back-bone. It emphasizes on Hardware elements, Computation requirements when the solution covers huge scope of medical problems at the mega scales across wide areas. This chapter discusses subsystems of the solution, that include Smart Phones, Computation Engines, High End Transportation Systems, Multi-Specialty Hospitals, Smart Phones/Digital Personal Assistants used by Medical Practitioners. Discusses on the accuracies, bandwidth requirements and latencies present in the systems, also emphasizes on the required accuracies as the problem area is Human Life. To address the challenges that arises when the solution gets high degree of maturity, this chapter proposes review of the current day protocols in the systems. Also proposes to integrate intelligent applications and different eco-systems like Big Data, Data Analytics and Internet of Things, and best adaptability of these areas with Nano-technologies to result in increased average life time of humans.

1. INTRODUCTION

Technology became a must for human beings in many ways over last 50 years. Starting from micron nodes to today's very advanced nodes of nanometer (Nano Technology) scales, technology has been impacting human life to make it more and more safer and speed. Along with its software models, technology has been delivering so

DOI: 10.4018/978-1-5225-1002-4.ch001

much value proposition in Computational Mathematics for all engineering fields, Medical Innovation, Educational Research, Defense Organizations, Automobiles, Mass Communications, Consumer Electronics. And especially in last decade electronics became a social need in the form of mobile devices. These mobile devices are embedding much computation power into it adding intelligence day by day. This added intelligence will help people to improve the productivity in multi fold.

This chapter, gives a hypothesis of Mobile Health Care, that means how a mobile device can be best used for the taking care of our health. And all the sub-systems involved into it from a preliminary view to high-end application usage.

In a simple view of this system, each user of mobile phone is connected with a health care center for immediate medical treatment and first aid. But there are multiple complex sub-systems take part in making it real.

This has been in practice in a very minimal level as pharmacy people keep enquiring us if we need any general medicine for seasonal diseases like cold and cough and also the regular medicine which we keep using as per prescription. Same model can be used for little more complex medical problems with the request initiated from an end user in the usage model. As per the criticality of the situations, medical conditions either first aid can be given or respective specialist can visit the patient with automated means of message processing systems.

2. HIGH LEVEL VIEW OF THE SOLUTION

Figure 1 is the pictorial view of the Mobile Health Care System, which shows all sub-systems, groups participating in the model. Each system on its own is again a complex system which needs accuracy and guaranteed service delivery model.

The system can be viewed as below:

1. End Users
2. High End Servers sitting cloud
3. Physicians and Hospitals
4. Mobile Services connected to hospitals or groups of hospitals.

End Users

All individuals who generates the requests for consulting services on different health problems. The requests either can be generated manually by the user or automatically by the sensors embedded into the mobile devices they carry. The sensors and respective intelligence embedded into the devices will continuously monitor dif-

Figure 1. System level view of the solution

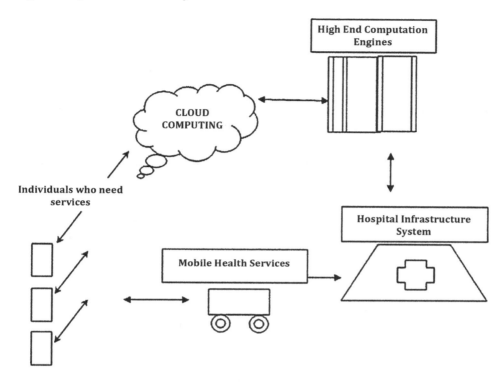

ferent health parameters of the individual and warn the user to consider for visiting a doctor. The software applications running on the mobile devices will process the collected data and send consulting signals to the master controller.

High End Servers

This is the place where high computation engine process the data received from the end user and find out the hospital or network of hospitals where the requests can be services. These engines will keep track of huge amount of data of all the people falling under its visibility. There can be multiple Clouds in the system to cater the requirements of all areas in a state according to the population. All the requests coming from different mobile devices are collected, stored and processed in this building block. This system needs high accuracy in delivery of the services. For enabling this guaranteed delivery, it also receives, stores the data from different hospitals in the area it covers. This is for ensuring the availability of respective specialists corresponding to a problem noticed from certain areas. High End Computation Engines sitting in the clouds, continuously monitors all the incoming lines from end user and also from hospitals. Along with hospitals, it also has to manage the Health Vehicles data and co-ordinate with specialists available with a particular vehicle.

Physicians and Hospitals

This block includes all the hospitals participating in the mobile health care. For this all the hospitals should be upgraded with the required facilities, Hardware and Software systems to enable the mobile health care services. All doctors should carry the mobile device which is enabled with required software. The doctors can communicate with applications running on the high-end servers for taking required actions-either he can accept the call from the cloud and immediately take one mobile-vehicle and attend the patient with in the safe time. Along with the existing health care models, all hospitals need to support the mobile care by dedicating the required resources.

Mobile Health Services

This block includes the ambulance services, mobile ICUs with specialists. This ensures immediate treatment to be started for a patient. This blocks integrates the multi-specialty services, first-aid, specialist consulting services for all kinds of emergency and critical care.

On top of all these building blocks of the said Mobile Health Care System, all the devices in those are having well defined intelligence for certain services like parameter measurement of 'N' number of health conditions, data extraction from the numbers measures, analysis of the extracted data, giving a brief based on the analysis done, and talk to corresponding specialists and try to bring up an environment where the patient can be started taking defined treatment. This involved all the existing subjects like- SW Engineering, Electronics Involved in each of the device, Networking of all the medical devices along with the mobile an individual carry, Data Analytics, Internet of Things.

3. DETAILED DESCRIPTION OF THE SUB-SYSTEMS

The following sections will give more details on the hardware present in each building block of the solution.

Mobile Devices

The devices which an individual carry can better be used to text, call or video conferencing with the nearby health care center in the simplest form of the solution. In addition to that, the devices can integrate different biometric sensors into it for collecting the continuous samples of health parameters like, Blood Pressure, Rate of the Heart Beat etc. We also have smart wearable devices which can replace the mobiles we use today. We also can integrate or connect different PDA (Personal Digital Assistants) which embed sensors to do more measurements like Sugar Levels in blood, Complete Blood Picture and any other new bio-metric measurements with the mobiles where health care applications are running. All these electronics devices integrated with the sensors, will be Wi-Fi enabled or also can communicate with our mobile via Blue Tooth interfaces for transferring the measured raw data. These data are collected by the mobile devices registered in the Mobile Health Care Solution and there its converted into a manageable data structure for communicating with other sub-systems of the solution.

Figure 2 shows sample images to describe on integration of sensors into mobile devices, PDAs which in turn can connected with mobiles without wires.

Figure 2. Bio sensors integrated with mobile devices

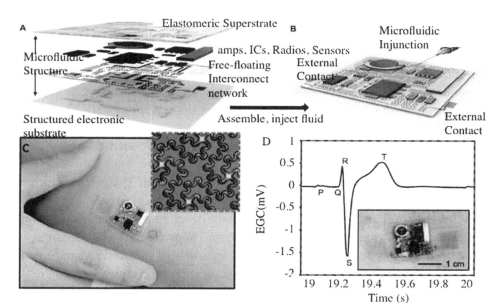

Likewise, sensors to monitor continuous the health conditions of individuals will be integrated into the mobile devices and the health care applications running in mobile processors, will collect, process and construct the LSD (Life Saving Data) and share with the solution. On receiving this data, Medical Assistants will observe the parameters, coordinate with the specialists and signal the ambulance systems in emergency cases, or directly interact with the individual for knowing further information and give medical advice appropriately. If not the Ambulance Systems can automatically reach the point of action and give first aid and brings to the hospitals.

High End Servers

As this solution need to process and route the service requests, Life Saving Data Structures with high degree of accuracies and speed, this Sub-System in the solution (High End Servers) need to provide high throughput and computing density along with built-in virtualization and extreme scalability. These includes highly efficient platforms for deploying large-scale, mission-critical applications. This versatility, along with powerful, bundled virtualization capabilities, makes them an ideal platform on which to consolidate large numbers of applications and databases.

As this sub-system is in the supply chain of a health care solution, these must satisfy requirements of Reliability, Availability, and Serviceability characteristics that make high service levels possible. Delivering RAS capabilities means much more than just having reliable components. It includes a combination of hardware and software features combined with advanced, integrated management and monitoring.

The servers provide an optimal solution for all database workloads, ranging from scan-intensive, complex data types, to highly concurrent online transaction processing applications. This on line processing of the transactions incurred in the solution also is a feature for addressing all financial part of the service model.

Mobile Devices Usage by Physicians and in Hospitals

The use of mobile devices by health care professionals (HCPs) has transformed many aspects of clinical practice. Mobile devices have become commonplace in health care settings, leading to rapid growth in the development of medical software applications (apps) for these platforms. Numerous apps are now available to assist HCPs with many important tasks, such as: information and time management; health record maintenance and access; communications and consulting; reference and information gathering; patient management and monitoring; clinical decision-making; and medical education and training.

Mobile devices and apps provide many benefits for HCPs, perhaps most significantly increased access to point-of-care tools, which has been shown to support better clinical decision-making and improved patient outcomes. However, some HCPs remain reluctant to adopt their use. Despite the benefits they offer, better standards and validation practices regarding mobile medical apps need to be established to ensure the proper use and integration of these increasingly sophisticated tools into medical practice. These measures will raise the barrier for entry into the medical app market, increasing the quality and safety of the apps currently available for use by HCPs.

Health Care Professions will use the advanced smart phones for managing the information they have for conducting their daily duties, time, for maintaining the Electronics Health Records, Electronic Medical Records for ease in accessing and storing them. And also they can use for scanning, sending, texting, encoding, audio and video conferencing with all required stake holders in the solution. Even Health Care Professionals will use these PDA (Personal Digital Assistants) for their reference study purposes for their personal development which in turn will help in better services to the point of actions.

Different usages of the PDA devices in hospitals are briefed below.

- **Information Management**: Physicians will make use of the PDA devices for writing and dictating notes, recording audio, taking photographs, organize information and images, for reading the reference books and also for accessing the services provided in clouds.
- **Time Management**: The devices are useful for physicians to schedule appointments, meetings and record the schedules. There can be apps developed for automating these tasks also, based on the categorization of the requests coming from individuals and also based on the type of the lifesaving data.
- **Records Maintenance and Access**: PDA are used for accessing Electronics Health Records (EHR) and Electronic Medical Records (EMR). The records cane be scanned images, scan reports, ECH reports, CT and MRI Scan Film records etc. Physicians can use the PDAs to coding of their medical notes on these electronic records for improvement purposes. And also they can use it for prescribing electronically on these records so that the newly generated records can be used in this solution in multifold.
- **Consulting and communicating the advices**: Physicians can use the PDA devices for voice, video calling with other specialists for discussing on certain issues on patients or, medical conditions. Even they can conduct international audio and video conferencing on chief advices of critical care conditions. Different applications running on these devices enable multimedia messaging, social networking in doctor's communities etc.

- **Reference Gathering and Educational purposes**: PDAs are also useful on educational purposes for continuous improvement of their skills and knowledge by managing the medical text books, journals, medical literature, keep referring to the research portals on their interesting domains, Drug reference guides and also news on their related topics can be tracked very efficiently by the physicians.
- **Clinical Decision-Making**: PDAs assists physicians in clinical decision support systems, treatment guidelines, diseases diagnosis aids, medical calculations, laboratory tests ordering, interpretation of the test results etc.
- **Patient Monitoring**: Monitoring patient's health, location, rehabilitation, collecting the clinical data, continuous monitoring of different parameters of patient health conditions.
- **Medical Education and Training**: Medical practisoners can continue their research programs or higher-education by efficiently using these Digital Devices. Conduct certain case studies. He can take assessment tests. Work on different surgical simulations when the problems are in very sensitive organs like heart or brains.

Mobile Health Care Systems

The current ambulance systems are a best example in the simplest view of the solution. Not only the immediate lifesaving medicines and first-aid services, this mobile system services are based on the service request type, and emergency conditions of the point of actions etc. Starting from first aid this system provides multi-specialty medical services.

Figure 3 can give brief on how ambulances can be integrated with all advanced lifesaving facilities of Intensive Care Units (ICUs) and be helpful for critical care conditions of the patients. Based on the services requests generated by the point of actions can exactly route to the very much required medical advisors automatically and in no time or allowable safer time periods, these advanced ambulances can come down to the point of actions and start giving treatment so that the patient survives.

4. PROBLEMS ASSOCIATED WITH THE SYSTEM

First of all, the points, the said system is going to be a player where "Human Life" is being to be main aspect of business. Given that fact, it is very much important to understand different limitations and bounded parameters of different electronics components participating in the solution. Major and known limitations of the

Figure 3. Transportation systems where reaching point of action is difficult

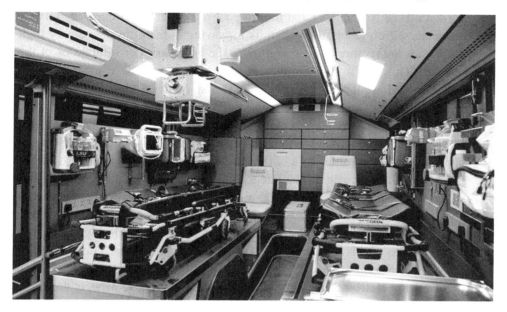

current day technologies are Limited Bandwidths, Security Features, Quality of Services, Device Power.

Along with the limitations of technologies, limitations imposed by current infrastructure which is going to fit in the solution in medical services is also important.

Below is the list of limitations of technology:

1. **Design Difference between Specification to Implementation**: +/- 5% of the tolerance in the design implementation to design specifications is going to play a major consideration while designing the sub-systems of the solution. All services must be designed with this deviation in consideration with mobile health care solution. There can be errors incurred into Life Saving Data while in air between the sub-systems.

2. **Probability of Errors Injected in to Data:** As the basic back-bone of the solution is wire-less technologies, there is always a probability of errors injected into the Life Saving Data Structure in air or within the electronic components of the sub-systems of solution. Each and every protocol will have this provision in definition itself, by making use of which the electronic components can be designed to limit the errors to very minimal. There must be error detecting and correcting algorithms to be implemented in each component of the sub-systems by making use of the protocol provisions.

3. **Limited Bandwidth in Data Communication**: All systems will be functioning with fixed frequencies that in turn pose a limitation in delays in delivery of services. But, given this system is for saving human life where very high accuracies are required, this can impose the boundaries or limitations of the services. This means, for example a patient who got cardiac arrest may not be given lifesaving guaranteed services in the moment of occurrence. Because the inaccuracies in all the involving systems in the above pictorial view are additive in nature, and hence it may take its own time for rendering the defined services and result in known delays. Because of this limitation, the solution needs to define the timeliness of the delivery of the services accordingly.

4. **Data Security:** Security of the integrity of the data is another concern in this solution. Because, it imposes a lot of issues when the solution gets maturity and start providing the services to a wider area networks. In this case, the basic data structures and SW Elements need to be defined with high degree of robustness to avoids security issues of the Life Saving Data. There are QOS (Quality of Services) aspects added in definition of all the protocols which involved in electronic components in the solution. These aspects are to be taken into consideration in defining the services, service limitations, services boundaries that results in high degree of security. Data Encryption, Decryption, 128-bit Security Keys should be implemented in handling the data integrity part of the solution.

All the above issues have to be mitigated in defining the solution.

5. **Infrastructure Facilities**: In addition to above technological limitations, there are few more problems associated with solution implementation. As the solution integrates multiple stake holders or sub-systems, current day infrastructure also imposes a problem here. Say, at highest degree of solution maturity, we need highly sophisticated transportation networks purely dedicated for these services. For example, an ambulance with high-en technology need to reach to point of service delivery within a stipulated time as per definition of the service.

6. **People Awareness**: For best utilization of the services of the solution, people also need to be knowledgeable to some extent. They have to be in a position to understand the steps and people involved in the system so that they provide necessary support. When there are multiple sensors integrated (we are going to discuss on sensors in next sections) into the mobile device, the individual need to understand how to make use of them. Though there are easy-to-understand human interface devices are defined, individuals should have minimum levels of technology awareness for best services. For this, governments have to work

towards 100% literacy among societies. At that juncture, this kind of solutions gain huge utilization factor.

5. SOLUTIONS FOR ABOVE PROBLEMS

This author had discussed the problems associated with the solution in above section and also tried to give solution while discussing the problems. When the system gets improvised over the period, these inaccuracies of tolerance, delays, data securities, bandwidth requirements can be avoided by mitigating them in design of every level of the sub-systems in the solution.

When we think of mitigating them, we should have a strong foundation in definition of the service primitives. Different stake holders from core medical researchers, marketing people, technology developers, Software Developers have to work on a common platform. This common platform has to be defined in an open source model and layered approach.

If we understand more on mitigating above problems and solutions into the mobile health care application of cloud computing, the author coins below terms that need to be addresses with more attention.

New Life Saving Data

The data which is generated, communicated, processed, serviced with this mobile health care solution has to be very robust enough that caters very wider life-span of the solution and services. Just like other Audio, Video and Text Data Type, this data has to be defines as a New Life Saving Data (LSD) and this should be well defined with all possible variations in the data in accordance with all possible health care services. Meaning, there should be a high-level data structure that addresses all kinds of general outpatient, emergency, critical care services required for all kinds of diseases, medical emergencies, accidents etc., This single new data structure keeps improvised over the period when many of medical services are brought under this solution. This way, all the Software, Hardware and System developers should be in sync to define the new data structure and deliver models, communication channels and services definition in exiting satellite communication.

All variations of the data structures should be defined by considering all the characteristics and parameters of all the medical emergencies, like different diseases, accidents, critical care requirements, allergies and general health problems. This set of defined packets can be categorized accordingly the allowable latencies in the treatments.

Irrespective of the data-type definition, end of the day this data is going to be transmitted and received over the wire-less and wired interfaces with in the solution. For this reason, the current protocols like Internet Protocol (IP), Wireless Lan Protocol (802.11), PCI Express Protocol (PCIe) need to be thoroughly analyzed and re-framed to fit in the parameters of this New Life Saving Data structures to cater needs of all medical problems, all wider area networks.

Quality of Services (QoS)

This solution will not compromise on the Quality of Services. Every request from any corner of the defined Safe Area of the solution must be communicated and given common resources for accurate and speed transfer of the Life Saving Data. In one abstractions (Open System Interface (OSI) Reference Model) all electronics systems generally designed into a layered architecture and each layer will have its own quality of services. All the existing designed will have to be re-visited and the respective functionality of each layer at each level in the solution should consider the LSD Type and its attached QOS Definition also at the very root level of the data types and communication model of the same.

Not only at the protocol level of the communication, the QOS aspects at each sub-system High-End Servers, Mobiles, Hospitals, Transport Means should be defined accordingly and ensure the delivery of the services with respect to the LSD Data Packets.

Internet of Things

Just like we connected to rest of our colleagues, known business connections, friend's circles, relatives and all known people every electronic gadget also gets connected to many other devices used by us. Every chord of this connectivity results in a specialized solution for solving different problems that human faces or provides a luxury of computation power to different data that humans need to know. Internet of things is becoming a new standard for smart cities, smart buildings, smart transportation, smart energy, smart industries, smart health and all together smart living. Application I.O.T can energize the Mobile Health Care Solution in a level beyond current imagination (Figure 4).

Smart Health: I.O.T

With I.O.T Eco System in place, all the electronic gadgets not necessarily the smart phones will have a communication channel and can accommodate future enhancements of the solution in current focus of this chapter. The Electronic Gadgets em-

Figure 4. Applications of internet of things

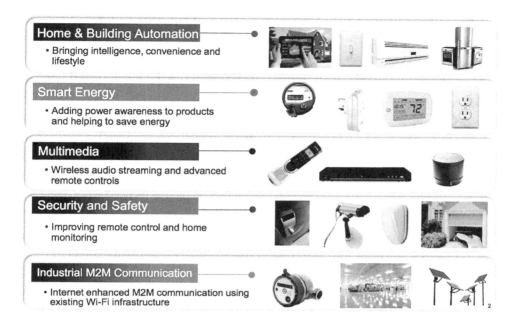

beds various Bio Metric Sensors with defined intelligence with their SW models will generate more quality medical data of the person that it is carried by and can pass of those data structures to local master command center where it can further be processed by and do take necessarily actions as required by the received Life Saving Data structure. It will co-ordinate with other sub-systems that are Advanced Ambulance Systems, Multi-Specialty Hospital Systems, Advanced Health Care Professionals in a regular programmable interval. The programmable intervals are also derived from the statistical data analysis of the services rendered and health patterns of the particular areas.

Eco System of Internet of Things in mind, we can best visualize the maturity levels of the Mobile Health Care solution with the advanced developments happening in the field of Biosensors and their integration into medical devices. We can propose, the integration of these Biosensors and devices which integrates these sensors with today's smart phones with the I.O.T as back bone of the networking of all the devices.

Biosensor Device

The diagram in Figure 5 explains the basic principle in the functionality of the Biosensors.

Figure 5. Basic principle of biosensor

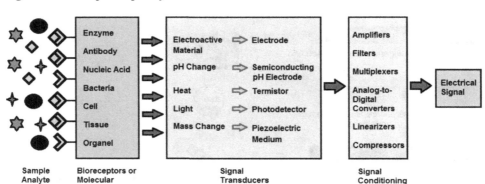

| Sample Analyte | Bioreceptors or Molecular Recognizers | Signal Transducers | Signal Conditioning Circuits |

As shown in above diagram, Biosensor Device is an analytical device that converts biological reactions into measurable signals like an electrical signal which is proportional to Target Analyte concentration in the input samples. A typical biosensor consists of two elements: biological sensing element in recognition layer and a transducer for the detection of Target Analyte concentration. Biological reaction takes place in close contact with the Transducer to ensure that most of the biological reaction is detected. A third element reference can be added along with the two elements which produce a small reference signal which can be an electrical or light signal. This signal serves as a control parameter for the representation of the observations. These observations help to decide on certain interpretations of health conditions and helps to take all necessary medical supporting actions.

Different Target Analytes which are studied with the biosensors in the Health Domain include for example an enzyme, an antibody, or a microorganism present in human body cells or blood samples.

The signal processing elements shown in the diagram are embedded in the Hardware portions of the smart phones which runs certain computational algorithms with a well-defined Software (or programming model). Both of these Software and Hardware elements are tightly coupled with a High Performance, High Speed Embedded Microprocessors sitting in the final electronic product.

As silicon-based chips are functional on the principles of materials science, biosensor transducers are additionally subject to biological principles. The target analyte in above diagram connected to an electronic element.

With the above explanation, we can define a biosensor as a biosensor is a self-contained integrated device, which is capable of providing specific quantitative or semi-quantitative analytical information using a biological recognition element (biochemical receptor) which is retained in direct spatial contact with an electrochemical transduction element. The first of its kind biosensor was developed in 1962 by Clark and Lyon as an „enzyme electrode, for the measurement of glucose levels in blood samples.

Taking above emphasis the Biosensor principle can be represented by Figure 6 with more details.

As per the advancements in the Transducer and in turn Biosensor technologies, the sensors can be implanted into human body in different places with a robust communication model to integrate with the Smart Phones. These biosensors are functionally useful for measuring different health parameters of the individuals who carry or implants those devices, and share the generated data with the Smart Phone in regular intervals. The Decision Making algorithms keep running in the smart phones will keep generating the necessary commands or data structures. These are the data structures which we have discussed as Life Saving Data Types.

Biosensor Signal Detection Methods

Below is a short list of some of the detection methods used in biosensors. The advantages and disadvantages can be point of importance for using these methods for suitability of adapting the method in our Health Care Solution. In our solution, main point we look at if the possibility of the miniaturization of the sensor technology.

- **Amperometry** is operated at a given applied potential between the working electrode and the reference electrode, and the generated signal is correlated

Figure 6. Biosensor components

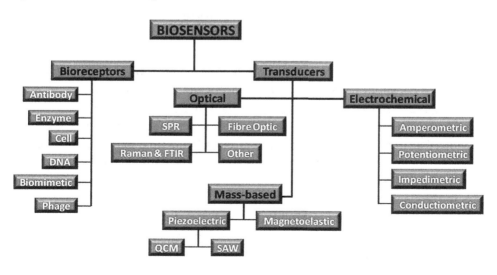

with the concentration of target compounds. In the amperometric detection, the current signal is generated as a function of the reduction or oxidation of an electro-active product on the surface of a working electrode.

- **Conductometry** is a technique depending on the conductivity change in the solution due to the production or consumption of ions, for example, by the metabolic activity of microorganisms. The measurement of conductance can be fast and sensitive, making conductometric microbial biosensors very attractive. Such biosensors are suitable for miniaturization since they require no reference electrode in the system.
- **Potentiometry** involves the measurement of the potential difference between the working electrode and the reference electrode which is dependent on concentration-related behavior. The transducer employed in the potentiometric technique is usually a gas-sensing electrode or an ion-selective electrode. The sensitivity and selectivity of potentiometric biosensor are outstanding due to the species-selective working electrode used in the system. However, a stable and accurate reference electrode is required.

When the scope of the medical problems assisted with this solution becomes wider and area of service delivery is wider, there will be huge amount of data generated in the solution. The processing of this huge amount of data becomes a tedious task when we think of the required accuracies, security and guaranteed delivery of the service. This problem can be better answered with the application of upcoming area of Big Data and Data Analytics in data processing. And we also have high computation engines sitting in clouds for helping us in solving this problem.

Smart Phones (PDAs) Where the Service Requests Are Generated from Individuals

These electronics gadgets must be designed for functioning with very low power requirements, so that battery life can be extended, so that no single case will miss the services because of drained battery in the gadget. Not only this, the data communication model needs re-definition for this to happen. This means, now all the data which is being transmitted from each electronics gadget will either be an isochronous data or bulk data. Meaning, isochronous being time sensitive, it will either be audio or video data and bulk being some kind of text files. And all these data types are having its own delivery models and guaranteed bandwidth allocations in from the SW and HW point of views.

But when we integrate the Mobile Health Care, systems will be re-visited for defining all the data transfer models from considering a new data type which is a Life Saving Data. Though it is Isochronous/ Bulk Type in nature, all together it is going to be a new data type from HW and SW stand point. The delivery models, arbitration of the common resources in this solution must be re-defined and tuned for addressing the new requirements of this Life Saving Data. Not only the new Data Type definition, re-definition of the existing communications systems, but also the Transport Means need to be reviewed and there must be a dedicated Transport Road Ways with good quality for safer and speeder mobility of the patients where next level of critical care is delivered to him.

In the hardware level implementations every protocol has definitions of Device Classes, QoS Models, Transaction Types etc., attributes into it. This special Life Saving Data structures should be treated and consider those provisions and can solve inaccuracies, delays etc in existing frame-works.

Data Analytics and Big Data

In comparison to products, services and physical means of business, present age can be treated as age of Digital Data. All the business starting with the very preliminary form of requirements are taking shape of the in Digital Data. Every second humans generating huge amount of data in the digital form and using that for correlation, populating the required information out from millions of bytes of digital data. This area is coming up as Data Analytics where Software Engineers are trying to abstract all the truths, myths into a set of data structures so that they can easily store, retrieve, process and run their analysis algorithms to bring out conclusions based on the numbers residing in the digital data.

The same can equally applies to our Mobile Health Care Solution in its novel version where huge amount of Life Saving Data needs high speed processing to bring out immediate medical solutions of any patient in any area in a predefined boundary. The same solution can recursively be applied to all defined bounded areas and cover entire area of interest, let us say City, Town, Village, District, State in an ideal level even entire nation can be covered with the solution.

6. FUTURE SCOPE

The advanced technologies like Internet of Things, Machine Intelligence, Artificial Intelligence, Robotics, Bi Data and Data Analytics play a major role when the solution gets matured to a level where the individuals who face any health issues will automatically route to the specialty treatment centers using this solution in well before the allowable safe time. At its high degree of maturity, the solution ultimately is going to reduce sudden deaths of human beings and in effect increases the average life time of humans. The solution at its maturity will drastically improves the healthy and quality life of humans. At its high degree of maturity, many biosensors with accessible, reliable, well defined machine intelligence can be integrated with today's mart phone in miniaturized way. Even different medical hand held devices can best be integrated with hand held smart phones in a well-defined communication channels.

7. CONCLUSION

Given today's advancements in miniaturization of the devices, high degree of integration of computing power, social penetration of mobile devices and different applications available, all together a sophisticated and efficient health care systems can be built around these technologies. This integration of all the aspects of Health Related Matters of human beings results in the best and in time diagnosis, accurate medical treatments, world class specialty medical and surgical services. With the focus of further improvements in medical procedures, Theory of Genes Decoding and Encoding, and their integration of next generation systems like High Density Computing, Robotics, Internet of Things, Data Analytics etc., will result in sophisticated health management and that in turn results in increasing the average life span of humans.

ADDITIONAL READING

Introduction to Biosensors. (n.d.). Retrieved from www.sirebi.org

Yoo, E.-H., & Lee, S.-Y. (2010). Glucose biosensors: An overview of use in clinical practice. *Sensors (Basel, Switzerland), 10,* 4558–4576. doi:10.3390/s100504558

Chapter 2
Cloud Based Wireless Infrastructure for Health Monitoring

Ajay Chaudhary
Indian Institute of Technology Roorkee, India

Sateesh Kumar Peddoju
Indian Institute of Technology Roorkee, India

Suresh Kumar Peddoju
Kakatiya Institute of Technology and Science, India

ABSTRACT

The wireless infrastructure based devices can collect data for long period of time even with a tiny power source as they perform specific function of collection of health related data and sending to gateways. The sensing data of healthcare monitoring consumes low power but they had limited computation power to process this data, where the cloud computing plays a vital role and compliment the loophole of wireless infrastructure based systems. In cloud computing with its immense computation power for easily deployment of healthcare monitoring algorithms and helps to process sensed data. As these two technologies did great jobs in their respective fields a conflate framework of these two technologies may lead to a great architecture for healthcare applications. This chapter reviews complete state-of-the-art and several use cases related to healthcare monitoring using different wireless infrastructure and adapting cloud based technologies in providing the healthcare services.

DOI: 10.4018/978-1-5225-1002-4.ch002

INTRODUCTION

World Health Organization (WHO, 2015b) defined several diseases and their cure based on age, gender, etc. Due to modern lifestyle and food habits, it is not easy to categorize any disease in a particular age group or gender, but still some diseases occur with time, and they need to manage accordingly. Several diseases like hypertension, cancer, diabetes, respiratory infections, road injuries, disability, and heart disease are leading to cause of deaths (WHO, 2015a). Several other diseases like asthma, stress and obesity are the secondary cause and leading to other diseases. Further, there are exceptional cases like children, disabled people, and elderly people need additional care. There are hundreds of diseases present worldwide. Some are zone specific other are commonly prevalent diseases. If proper treatment is available, many lives can be saved.

Traditional Healthcare Systems

The traditional healthcare system is based on two basic principles i.e. either doctor has to visit the patient for treatment or patient has to go to the medical practitioner, hospital, clinic, and/or day care center. There is no other method of treatment available to treat illness or severe disease effectively. In traditional health care system if patient's condition is critical then he/she may be admitted to hospital but even for a routine checkup like blood pressure patient need to visit a doctor or record it at home manually and report the same to the doctor. There is no automated system which can monitor all vital signs of patients automatically and report them to the doctor as and when needed or a doctor can check the current vital statistics of the patient and regulate the treatment in real time. The traditional healthcare management scenario is changing drastically with the emergence of prominent infrastructures including cloud and wireless networks like Wireless Sensor Network (WSN) or Body Sensor Network (BSN). Mobile and pervasive computing (MPC) have become the third wave of the world information industry after the computer and the Internet. Individually these technologies contribute exhaustively for the development of general purpose applications by providing better and cost effective sensing and computation power. As the wireless infrastructure based technologies make a significant contribution in the broad range of areas including forest -fire monitoring, weather- forecasting, structural health monitoring, smart cities, smart homes and smart offices to health and elderly monitoring. On the other hand, the cloud plays a vital role in its services that make a computation or storage of massive data with ease, fast and minimal cost.

The wireless infrastructure elements like WSN, BSN, and MPC enhanced real remote sensing benefits due to its infrastructure-less deployments, capabilities to sense data at remote areas and ability to communicate with each other without any wires. Also, the wireless infrastructure based devices can collect data for a long duration even with a little power source as they perform a particular function of a collection of data and sending to gateways. The running of sophisticated health monitoring algorithms or any similar algorithms on massive datasets on these small devices is not feasible. Since they have a limited computation power and the cloud computing plays a vital role and compliments the processing of wireless infrastructure based systems. In cloud computing with its "infinite" computation power, these algorithms can be easily deployed and run. Keeping in view of the importance of these two technologies, WSN and Cloud, a conflate framework of these two technologies may lead to a great architecture for healthcare applications. It would be possible to implement a healthcare system that can provide the healthcare services to a person by encapsulating the underneath constraints of location, time, accessibility and availability. The system may be able to provide adequate healthcare facility to everyone across the globe without any timing or geographical constraints. This leads to a quality healthcare system across the world. A patient at the remote location with proper deployment of such combined framework of sensor and cloud may bring a quality treatment from the best doctor in the world without visiting him in person.

Basics of Wireless Infrastructure

1. Concept

The Wireless sensor network consists of an infrastructure-less system in which nodes are deployed in the range from tens to thousands without any physical link and layout. The various sensor nodes can be deployed over the body in a non-invasive fashion as shown in Figure 1 and they must not interfere with the daily life of the patients i.e. there should not be any hindrance due to the sensor node or patient need to do some lifestyle modification in order to get adapted as per sensor node requirements. Based on various disease types, these sensor nodes can collect the data and same data is transferred over the network to the doctor for examination with reports.

2. Applications

They are deployed everywhere from the battlefield to forest fire detection, from structural health monitoring to human health monitoring, from smart cities to landslide monitoring, and from air quality monitoring to water quality monitoring. Even it is widely used in the critical process of chemical reaction monitoring and to control reactions in nuclear power plants. The wireless sensors are also widely used in habitat monitoring, biodiversity monitoring, active volcano monitoring,

Figure 1. Deployment of various sensor nodes on body

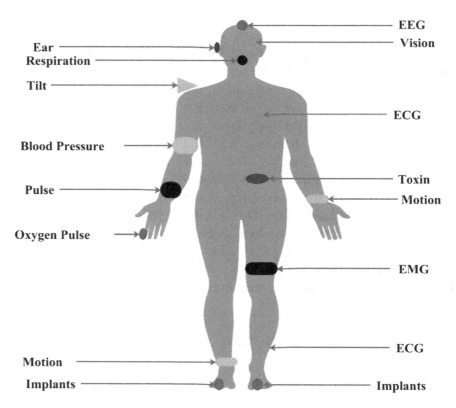

underground mine monitoring like coal mines and precision agriculture. The sensor networks or its variants like body sensor network are deployed almost everywhere we can think of. The most commonly used applications of WSN are (Libelium, 2015) E-Healthcare, Smart Cities, Smart Environment, Smart Water, Security and Emergencies, Logistics and Retail, Industrial Control, Domestic and Home Automation, and Defense and Military purpose.

3. Types of Sensors

The sensor nodes are deployed widely almost in all the fields base on their capacity to sense various parameters (Rakocevic, 2009) like pressure, motion (accelerometers), temperature sensors, humidity sensors, chemical sensors, biosensors, luminosity, gyroscope, gasses (CO_2, O_2), acoustic, GPS etc. Typical sensors and their importance is presented in the following Table 1.

Table 1. Typical list of sensors

S. No.	Sensor Type	Sensor Sub Type	Operations and functionality
1.	Pressure sensors	Piezoresistive pressure sensors	Piezoresistor are integrated into a membrane. Pressure or force applied directly to a member causing it to deform, hence pressure or force is measured.
2.		Capacitive pressure sensors	If pressure/force is applied to the sensor surface, causing a membrane to deflect resulting in capacitance to change and pressure or force is measured. It can measure pressure with great sensitivity but had high production cost.
3.	Accelerometers	Resistive and capacitive accelerometers	In these sensor devices, an elastic cantilever with an attached mass is usually used to measures relative change in speed of the object based on a change in resistance or capacitances. These are generally used to measures constant acceleration.
4.		Piezoelectric accelerometers	Piezoelectric accelerometers are based on the piezoelectric effect. In this, an electric charge is created when the sensing material is squeezed or strained.
5.	Temperature sensors	Electromechanical temperature sensors	It measures the temperature based on expanding and contracting properties of materials using a bi-metal thermostat.
6.		Resistive Temperature sensors	It measures the temperature based on a property of resistant changes with temperature.
7.	Humidity sensors	Capacitive RH Sensors	In a capacitive relative humidity (RH) sensor, humidity measures in term of change in dielectric constant which is directly proportional to relative humidity.
8.		Resistive Humidity Sensors	It measures humidity in term of resistance changes in the environment as resistance is inversely proportional to the environmental humidity. Resistive humidity sensors are small size, low cost, and are usable from remote locations.
9.	Gyroscope	Vibration Gyro Sensors	The piezoelectric transducer or silicon transducer based are sensors used to measures the orientation of the objects and/or rotation of the object.
10.	Image Sensor	active pixel sensor (CMOS)	It detects and conveys information in order to constitute an image by converting waves in signals.
11.	Light Sensor	Ambient Light Sensor (ALS)	It approximates the human eye response under a variety of light conditions.
12.	GPS	GPS	Devices have a base station which measures the position based on geostationary GPS satellites, at least, three satellite are required to measure exact position, work with high precision in outdoor environments.
13.	Acoustic, sound sensor	Microphone	Measure sound wave by converting them into signals.
14.	Blood Pressure Sensor	Sphygmomanometer Sensor	They measure systolic/diastolic blood pressure of the patient.
15.	Heartbeat rate monitoring sensor	Pulse sensor	Noninvasively monitors heart rate when placed over a fingertip of the patient.
16.	Proximity Sensor	Capacitive, IR or other type of sensors	Proximity sensors detect the presence of objects without physical contact. It had a large range of sensors such as inductive sensors, photoelectric sensors, magnetic sensors other than capacitive sensors, and IR sensors.
17.	Tactile Sensor	distributed capacitive tactile sensor	Measures the touch over the surface.

continued on following page

Table 1. Continued

S. No.	Sensor Type	Sensor Sub Type	Operations and functionality
18.	GSR - Sweating	Galvanic Skin Response (GSR) Sensor	The nervous system controls the sweat glands of the skin. The psychological changes directly reflect the changes in electrical conductance of the skin which is also known as galvanic skin response.
19.	Position Sensor	accelerometer	Using piezoelectric accelerometers.
20.	Blood Glucose sensor	Glucometer sensor	Glucometer is a medical device for determining the approximate concentration of glucose in the blood.
21.	muscle/ eletromyography sensor (EMG)	Muscle Sensor	Measuring muscle activation via electric potential referred to as electromyography (EMG).
22.	Electroencephalography (EEG)	EEG Sensor	It is used to monitor and record brain's spontaneous electrical activity over a period.
23.	Oxygen (spO2) sensor	Pulse Oximeter	The amount of oxygen saturation level present in blood is monitored using the non-invasive method.
24.	Speed sensor	Speed sensor	It detects the speed of an object. It measures the relative speed of the object.
25.	Airflow Sensor	Breathing Sensor	Measures the oxygen intake.
26.	electrocardiogram (ECG)	ECG (or EKG) sensor	Noninvasively monitor and record the electrical activity of the heart over the span of time and generate an electrocardiograph.
27.	ultrasound sensors	Ultrasonic transducers	Ultrasonic sensors transmit ultrasonic waves from its sensor head and again receives the ultrasonic waves reflected from an *object*.
28.	Chemical sensors	Piezoelectric chemical sensors	The piezoelectric effect is generated with a change in chemical composition of an environment.
29.		Ion-sensitive FET sensor	Ion concentration (such as pH) changes lead to a change in the flow of current through the transistors.
30.		Conductivity sensors	Interaction with certain gasses may result in a change in conductivity as a result; it detects chemical leakage.
31.	Biosensors	Biosensors	Used to detect the presence of bacteria, viruses, or molecules and molecular complexes like proteins, enzymes, antibodies, DNA, etc. for several applications. Biosensors are also to check effects of external environment on the body and measure presence of antibodies or enzymes etc.
32.	Radiation sensors	Geiger-Müller counter	Used to detect gamma and beta radiations, but certain models support alpha radiations also. It measures the presence of radiation level in the environment and alerts based on the threshold value.
33.		Quartz fiber dosimeter	Sensitive to gamma and X-ray but can also detect beta rays. It measures the presence of radiation level in the environment and alert based on the threshold value.

Basics of Cloud Computing

1. Definition

According to NIST, the definition of cloud computing is (Mell & Grance, 2011)

Cloud computing is a model for enabling ubiquitous, convenient, on-demand network access to a shared pool of configurable computing resources (e.g., networks, servers, storage, applications, and services) that can be rapidly provisioned and released with minimal management effort or service provider interaction.

This cloud model is composed of five essential characteristics, three service models, and four deployment models.

2. Essential Characteristics

The cloud computing environment must be able to provide at least some essential services which acts as a standard for cloud service providers. Also, there are many optional services which depend on vendors. These essential services are listed below (Mell & Grance, 2011):

1. **On-Demand Self-Service:** The system must be able to serve the requirements of the clients on the fly with no human involvement. It should be able to allocate resources for storage, compute power, network and other services based on client request in real time.
2. **Broad Network Access:** The cloud computing infrastructure must be widely accessed on the various platforms using the standard mechanism. It must support heterogeneous client platforms. A cloud computing resources must be accessible through smartphones, tablets, desktop PC and workstations or mainframe.
3. **Resource Pooling:** The computing resources must be shared among the clients and serve their requirements using multi-tenant model. It must be capable of assigning physical and virtual resources to the clients on the go; the resource can be reassigned dynamically to fulfill the demand of the customers.
4. **Rapid Elasticity:** Cloud must provide rapid elasticity to fulfill demands of user ranging from 1 machine to 1000 machines with easily scale up and scale down.
5. **Measured Service:** A metering capability should help to monitor all the resources used by the client and charge transparently. The resource utilization should be properly monitored, reported; there should also be a provision for auditing the metering services by a trusted third party.

3. Service Models

The cloud vendors provide different services to their clients. These services are categories as (Mell & Grance, 2011):

1. **Software as a Service (SaaS):** The cloud-based applications are provided by the cloud provider running on their infrastructure. The customer can access the application over the internet. There is no need to install and maintain them locally. The client can access using various interfaces like web, thin clients or through client's end program or API.
2. **Platform as a Service (PaaS):** The cloud-based development and testing platforms, operating systems, databases etc., are provided by the cloud provider to run client's applications. It makes the client hassle free in procuring the proprietary products, buying the licenses etc.
3. **Infrastructure as a Service (IaaS):** IaaS is a elastic and multi-tenant model in which the resources like computation power, storage and network owned and hosted by the provider are offered to the several clients on sharing basis.

4. Deployment Models

The most common deployment models of cloud are (Mell & Grance, 2011):

1. **Private Cloud:** Cloud deployed by the organization for its own use. The hardware may exist within or outside the organizations' physical premises and can be accessible from various offices of organization using VPN or other networks.
2. **Community Cloud:** This type of cloud infrastructure is sharable within community for common purpose such as specific mission, policy or requirements. It may be managed by specific organization within community or third party.
3. **Public Cloud:** The public cloud services are accessible to organizations or individuals on payment basis. It is helpful for renting services for specific project or during specific peak hours without any burden of procuring hardware.
4. **Hybrid Cloud:** This model of cloud infrastructure is having two or more models discussed above used together. For example, organizations can extend their resources using public or community cloud during test and development period along with its private cloud. The hybrid cloud provides flexibility to extend resources to fulfill resource demands during peak usage.

HEALTHCARE RESEARCH

This section presents the state-of-the-art in wireless infrastructures and cloud infrastructures independently through reviewing several existing research papers in the light of health care management.

Wireless Infrastructures in Healthcare

The Wireless sensor network or Body sensor network based devices are widely used to help patients suffering from Hypertension, cancer, diabetes, respiratory infections, Road injuries and disability, heart disease, asthma, stress, and obesity etc. in elders. WSN is widely used in the Child health care management of diseases such as asthma, cerebral palsy, autism, obesity, and overweight. Wireless sensor-based devices are also widely playing a vital role in disabilities management include visually, deaf etc., elderly care like Parkinson's disease and fall detections. Figure 2 indicates the general framework of the wireless infrastructures in healthcare.

Figure 2. Wireless infrastructures in healthcare monitoring

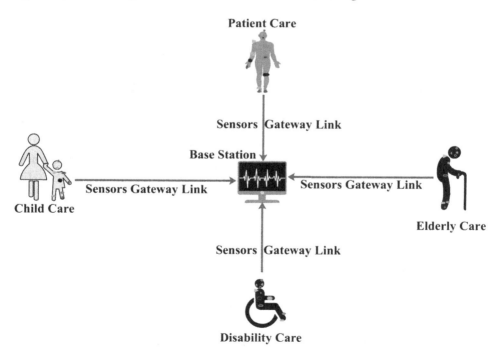

1. General Studies

There are several existing research papers published highlighting the role of wireless infrastructures on healthcare monitoring (Acampora, Cook, Rashidi, & Vasilakos, 2013; Alemdar & Ersoy, 2010; Orwat, Graefe, & Faulwasser, 2008; Pantelopoulos & Bourbakis, 2010; Uniyal & Raychoudhury, 2014; Varshney, 2007). Few papers are reviewed to understand the state-of-the-art in wireless infrastructures that contribute to healthcare.

Varshney (2007) discussed various aspects of pervasive healthcare such as health monitoring, data access, telemedicine and management of medical emergencies. The author emphasized the deployment and implementation aspects of various wireless network solutions like wireless LANs, ad hoc networks, and cellular or mobile networks in order to provide infrastructure for pervasive healthcare. The paper also emphasized on various aspects of pervasive healthcare including context awareness, reliability, autonomy and adaptiveness. Orwat et al. (2008) presented a comprehensive study on research reported during the period of 2002 to 2006. The study considered various parameters like present prototypes, case studies and pilot studies, clinical trials and systems that are already in routine. The study is also based on categories like project status, health care settings, user groups, improvement aims, and systems features (i.e., component types, data gathering, data transmission, systems functions). In addition, the paper covered a quantitative analysis based on deployment issues, organizational and personal issues, privacy and security issues and financial issues.

Pantelopoulos and Bourbakis (2010) performed an exhaustive study on wearable biosensor systems for health monitoring and also biosensors research & development advances. They compared implementations based on qualitative and quantitative features in order to categorize the current state-of-the-art in wearable biosensor solutions. They took parameters such as multi-parameter physiological sensing systems design, providing reliable vital signs measurements and incorporating real-time decision support for early detection of symptoms or context awareness and defined their maturity levels. Alemdar and Ersoy (2010) evaluated the benefits of wireless sensor technologies for patient healthcare and elderly healthcare, and how they get benefited from wireless sensor technologies in order to provide care at home. They classified systems based on acquiring and interpreting the context information for better deployment of WSN based architectures. They also suggested research paradigm of multi-modal sensors that cost low, energy-efficient and ad hoc deployment model of sensor networks for better medical care.

Acampora et al,(2013) categorized and classified the infrastructure and technologies in order to support the Ambient Intelligence (AmI) paradigm which empowers the people's capabilities of using digital environment which is sensitive, adaptive and responsive to the human needs, habits, gestures and even emotions. The AmI enables human-machine interaction pervasive, unobtrusive and seamless manner. The authors discussed the role of amI in healthcare domain and provided the necessary background for research community by examining infrastructure and technology requirements to achieve the vision of AmI. A set of existing applications of AmI in healthcare systems are also listed. Uniyal and Raychoudhury (2014) defined the classification system based on the diseases present in various gender and age groups respectively. The study presented the existing tools and techniques used in pervasive healthcare; based on major diseases in various age and gender groups. They also listed commercially available pervasive healthcare products and open challenges of pervasive healthcare base system.

2. Patient Care

The Wearable sensors are capable of monitoring the significant physiological be-haviors of patients including heart rate, blood pressure, body and skin temperature, oxygen saturation, respiration rate, and electrocardiogram. Such physiological symptoms can be monitored and reported using low-power sensors such as pulse oximetry, respiration rate, and temperature. Several authors (Morrison, 1997; Super, Groth, & Hook, 1994) reported triage protocols for emergency medical services for mass-casualty disasters monitoring. But on large scale mass causality, these protocols are inefficient and they lose their effectiveness as the number of victims increases. In such scenario, the portable, scalable and rapidly deployable body sensors and pervasive healthcare systems help to monitor physiological levels of large number of victims at the same time in the hospital and outside the hospital during move-ment from the site of causality to the hospital. These sensors keep track of record on vital signs of patients and help doctors to keep treatment ready even before the arrival of the patient to the hospital.

3. Elderly Care

At home care of elderly patients/persons need special attention. They face several challenges due to health, social, psychological status, and quality of life (Wood et al., 2008). Due to their age factor they are more vulnerable to the diseases like congestive heart failure, asthma, diabetes, Parkinson's disease, chronic obstructive pulmonary disease, and memory decline. these diseases tender great set of chal-lenges to the doctors in order to monitor and treat them. As discussed in traditional systems, either patients need to visit doctor or doctors need to visit patients. It will be really hard to manage the overall system as patients are restricted to stay in bed in order to record and monitor the signs. The wireless network based pervasive healthcare system helps to monitor the such signs in real-time without restricting the patient's movement and their daily routines. The some of the most common diseases are briefly presented below:

a. Fall-Detection

World Health Organization in its report of fall detection and prevention (WHO, 2007) stated that approximately 28-35% of people aged 65 and above fall each year while it is increased to 32-42% for those over 70 years of age. The frequency of falls increases with age and frailty level. The fall causes 20-30% of mild to severe injuries and one of the major reason of medical emergencies. Falls account for 40% of all injury deaths. The fall is a major issue for elderly care. The cause of falls increases with aging due to biological changes, as a result, there is a high incidence of falls and fall-related injuries (Igual, Medrano, & Plaza, 2013). The pervasive healthcare plays a vital role in preventing and detecting such falls related injuries; the studies carried out in this field are reported in the following sub-sections.

i. Context-Aware Systems

The context-aware systems detect fall based on sensors deployed in the environment. The patient need not wear any sensor. However, this type of system restricts the patient movement to the limited area only. There are several context-aware systems developed. Few (T. Lee & Mihailidis, 2005) used video sensing as an underlying source of input while other systems (Shaou-Gang, Pei-Hsu, & Chia-Yuan, 2006) are based on image processing using connected components labeling and feature extraction. (Vishwakarma, Mandal, & Sural, 2007) used feature extractions and rule-based detection method. In the same year, (Cucchiara, Prati, & Vezzani, 2007) used the tracking algorithm and histogram. In the year 2008, (Fu, Delbruck, Lichtsteiner, & Culurciello, 2008) used the tracking algorithm and temporal average of motion events; (Hazelhoff & Han, 2008) used the tracking algorithm and PCA-based feature extractions. In 2010, (Liu, Lee, & Lin, 2010) used image processing with the mean feature, feature extraction and K- nearest neighbor algorithm based detection while (Rimminen, Lindström, Linnavuo, & Sepponen, 2010) used the tracking algorithm and two-state Markov chain (falling, getting up). (Zhang, Tian, & Capezuti, 2012) usd the tracking algorithm and histogram to detect the fall. (Anderson et al., 2009) extracted the features such as centroid, height, major orientation of the body and then applied fuzzy logic based rules. (Williams, Ganesan, & Hanson, 2007) used distributed camera infrastructure in order to detect fall. (C.-W. Lin & Ling, 2007) developed a system that can be able to differentiate fall from other normal activity. (Diraco, Leone, & Siciliano, 2010) presented a method to detect the posture of fall. (Abu-Faraj, Akar, Assaf, Al-Qadiri, & Youssef, 2010) defined a system in which all detection and recovery are done using dynamic plantar pressure measurement.

ii. Wearable Sensors

Wearable sensor-based fall detection system requires the patients to wear sensors. In most of the applications, the victim need to wear accelerometer sensor. Acceleration data are collected during fall time using independent tri-axial accelerometers attached to different parts of the body. The Threshold Based Method (TBM) measures the velocity right from an initial contact with ground and measures the spatial direction of fall. (Lindemann, Hock, Stuber, Keck, & Becker, 2005) developed a TBM by placing the sensor behind the ear of patient and tested on young volunteers and elderly women. (J. Chen, Kwong, Chang, Luk, & Bajcsy, 2006) developed a TBM by placing the sensor on the waist and able to detect backward and sideways fall. (A. K. Bourke, O'Brien, & Lyons, 2007) developed a TBM by placing the sensor on trunk and thigh and able to detect forward falls, backward falls, lateral falls on left and right. (Kangas, Konttila, Lindgren, Winblad, & Timo, 2008) developed a TBM by placing the sensor on the waist, head and wrist to detect forward, backward and lateral falls. (Kangas et al., 2009) developed a TBM by placing the sensor on the waist and able to detect slipping, lateral fall, rolling out of bed. (Q. Li et al., 2009) developed a TBM by placing the sensor on chest and thigh and able to detect forward, backward, sideways and vertical falls even falling on stairs and against wall. (Bianchi, Redmond, Narayanan, Cerutti, & Lovell, 2010) developed a TBM by placing the sensor on the waist and able to detect Forward, backward and lateral falls. (Alan K. Bourke et al., 2010) developed a TBM by placing the sensor on the waist and able to detect Forward, backward and lateral falls left and right. (Lai, Chang, Chao, & Huang, 2011) developed a TBM by placing the sensor on the neck, hand, waist and foot, and able to detect forward, backward, rightward and leftward falls. (Bagala et al., 2012) developed a TBM by placing the sensor on lower back and able to detect forward, backward and sideway fall both in a real and outdoor environment. Cheng (Juan, Xiang, & Minfen, 2013) developed a TBM by placing the sensor on chest and thighs, and able to detected forward, backward, left sideway and right sideways.

b. The Paralysis Agitans or Parkinson's Disease

Yet, another most common disease affecting adult's health is a loss of body control resulting to Paralysis agitans, shaking palsy or more commonly known as Parkinson's disease (PD) which is a chronic and progressive movement disorder, meaning that symptoms continue and worsen over time. This disease affects the elderly men and women both. (Q. Lin, Zhang, Ni, Zhou, & Yu, 2012) developed a GPS-based pervasive healthcare platform for smart phones to provide personal assistance to elderly people whenever needed. It provides health support, safety assurance, and daily activities assistance. (LeMoyne, Coroian, & Mastroianni, 2009) quantified the Parkinson's disease characteristics using wireless 3D MEMS accelerometers and

(LeMoyne, Mastroianni, Cozza, Coroian, & Grundfest, 2010) also demonstrated that iPhone wireless accelerometer application can be used to quantify Parkinson's disease, even from thousand miles away. (Okuno, Yokoe, Fukawa, Sakoda, & Akazawa, 2007) measured the finger-tapping contact force for the quantitative diagnosis of Parkinson's disease. They used 3-axis piezoelectric element accelerometers and touch sensors made of thin stainless steel sheets. They developed a transfer function that determines the contact force during finger tapping phase. (Shima et al., 2008) developed a model to determine finger tapping for the quantitative diagnosis of Parkinson's disease by using the magnetic sensor. They used finger stiffness function in order to determine the finger tapping characteristics and they (Shima, Tsuji, Kandori, Yokoe, & Sakoda, 2009) also quantified and evaluated finger tapping movements for the assessment of motor function using log-linearized Gaussian mixture networks (LLGMNs) with magnetic sensors.

4. Disability Care

Patient's living with disability and their rehabilitation is another issue needed to be addressed. Pervasive healthcare systems play a vital role as the sensor network systems guide and assist the patients during their daily routines. The sensors monitor the signs and the surrounding conditions in order to assist the patient intelligently. These intelligent sensors monitor and record the vital signs for the long term as they assist the patient in real-time. The data collected by these sensors helps the trainer to decide the tailor-made training schedules for the patient and, as a result, the overall impact of the training increases manifolds. The traditional device is modified and embedded with state-of-the-art sensor technologies in order to use the capabilities of the sensor network and they are helping the patients instead of providing just support (Visintin, Barbeau, Korner-Bitensky, & Mayo, 1998). These sensor-enabled devices now play a vital role in navigation for visually challenged patients (Bohonos, Lee, Malik, Thai, & Manduchi, 2007; Coughlan & Manduchi, 2007). The researchers at the University of Florida developed Drishti navigation system which helps visually impaired and disabled persons to navigate in outdoor, based on GPS and speech assistant (Helal, Moore, & Ramachandran, 2001) and navigate both indoor and outdoor based on GPS and ultrasound tags (Ran, Helal, & Moore, 2004). Based on ultrasonic sensors, researchers developed systems which enables the patient's indoor movement and even allow them to play indoor games (Y.-B. Lee & Lee, 2009). Systems which guide the patients in outdoor environment also provides feedback about presence of obstacles on their way by mean of vibrations (Yu, Yoon, & Jeong, 2013). RFID-based systems are used to help a visually challenged person in order to help them to identify the bus (El Alamy, Lhaddad, Maalal, Taybi, & Salih-Alj,

2012) and provide indoor navigations (Ganz et al., 2012). There are several systems developed that provide remote control to the computer operations based on camera and mouse (Betke, Gips, & Fleming, 2002), voice assistance (Krasij, Pruehsner, & Enderle, 1999; Struijk, 2006), head movement (O. Takami, Irie, Kang, Ishimatsu, & Ochiai, 1996), head and eyeball movement (Osamu Takami, Morimoto, Ochiai, & Ishimatsu, 1995) and tilt sensor (Y.-L. Chen, 2001). Researchers developed a system for the remote control assistant for thermostat and door opener (Tartamella, Pruehsner, & Enderle, 1999), and household electronic item controller (Alecsandru, Pruehsner, & Enderle, 1999). The progression of the Parkinson Disease can be measured by the UPDRS (Unified Parkinson Disease Rating Scale) scale which is used to evaluate behaviorally and motor symptoms of Parkinson's disease. (Kupryjanow, Kunka, & Kostek, 2010) used Virtual-Touchpad (VTP), a multimodal interface, to determine the level of Parkinson Disease in the patients.

5. Child Care

The side effect of modern lifestyle on children is worsening their health profile and obesity is one of major diseases. Although there is vaccination schedule for newborn baby to help them fight with all major diseases like measles etc. but still in some diseases like Cerebral palsy in which child loses control and not able to control the body movement. These days' children also suffer from diseases that are meant for elders like sleep apnea, autism, BP, sugar, cancer etc. There is a major research focused on the Cerebral palsy assistance. There is childcare system developed by (Starida, Ganiatsas, Fotiadis, & Likas, 2003) keep an electronic record of child medicine history, Streamline doctors, and caretaker communication providing virtual collaborative space for the cooperation of healthcare professionals, delivering alerts and reminders etc. (McCann, Wang, Zheng, & Eccleston, 2012) developed an interactive questionnaire system for child care to determine the chronic pain without even visiting the doctors. The questionnaire information is analyzed and evaluated and then provided to the doctor in order to to assess the situation. (Chuah & DiBlasio, 2012) developed a smart phone-based autism social alert system that monitors the autistic children's behavior using embedded sensors in smart phones. They also used the environmental sensors in order to determine the environmental condition simultaneously in order determine the triggering factor for stereotypical behaviors of such children. (Pruette, Fadrowski, Bedra, & Finkelstein, 2013) developed a system to monitor the children with high BP using mobile BP tele-management system having three units; home unit, decision support server and care management site. The home unit has a wireless netbook and a BP sensor which record the BP. It maintaines a symptom diary, assess medication side effects, obtain BP, undergo hypertension education, and communicate with the decision support server.

CLOUD INFRASTRUCTURES IN HEALTHCARE

The cloud computing is an emerging computing paradigm that provides services to its customers through the web or app-based interfaces on the basis of pay per use. The cloud provider offers several advantages like metered services, scale up and scale down of resources, on demand services, customize architecture, software, and hardware, almost unlimited compute and storage space etc. The flexibility, always uptime and on-demand resources allocation open new avenues for the other sector like healthcare to use cloud computing-based solutions for its needs (Sultan, 2013). Figure 3 gives an overview of application of Cloud infrastructures in Healthcare monitoring.

In the USA, the patient/protected health information (PHI) and patient health record (PHR) must be stored at secure server location in order to meet the requirement of Health Insurance Portability and Accountability Act (HIPAA) (HIPPA, 1996) same will be applied to the cloud computing scenario.

Sultan (2013) presented a virtual environment using simulated e- Health pilot project implemented in London in order to demonstrate the potential advantages to the patients by using cloud services. The patient's personal health record (PHR) is kept in hospital in order to diagnosis and provide medical assistantship to the patients as and when required. The PHR has emerged as a patient-centric model of health information exchange. The PHR service helps to maintain patient's personal health data and allow the patient to create, manage and control his/her health information through a simple web-based interface which enables storage, retrieval and sharing of medical records among the concern doctors more efficient way. Microsoft Health Vault (microsoft, 2015) is a third party cloud based healthcare servicing system to maintain patient health records. (Ming, Shucheng, Yao, Kui, & Wenjing, 2012) presented a novel framework which enables secure sharing of PHR over the cloud computing

Figure 3. Cloud infrastructures in healthcare monitoring

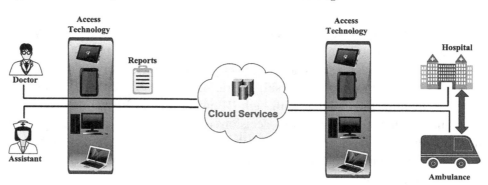

environment with the assumption that cloud service provider is trustworthy. They allow the patient to store their health record in encrypted format, they addressed the issues like key management and privacy, they used the attribute-based encryption (ABE) to encrypt the PHR data. They created a role to access the data of PHR and then granted the access based on attributes to these roles. They (M. Li, Yu, Ren, & Lou, 2010) also proposed a secure access to the cloud computing resources and PHR within cloud computing environment. They use attribute-based encryption (ABE) techniques to encrypt each patient's PHR data. In order to reduce the key distributions complexity, they divided the system into multiple security domains; each domain only caters the small set of users. In the security domain based method, they were able to provide each patient a maximum privacy of the medical records and they also reduced the key distribution complexity. There is a flexibility of revocation of roles and in emergencies, a break glass protocol is used to access patient PHR. (Shucheng, Cong, Kui, & Wenjing, 2010) suggested attribute-based encryption (KP-ABE) encryption technique in order to keep patient health information (PHI) securely over the cloud environment. Their security policy enables the data owner to delegate the compute intensive task to powerful cloud servers. This is necessary in order meet up the requirement of HIPAA (HIPPA, 1996).

The key aspect of the electronic healthcare applications is not only the ubiquitous availability but also their ability to integrate with social dynamics irrespective of cultural differences and individuals' preferences; it must be usable around the globe and accessible by the individuals irrespective of their residential locations. Keeping this aspect in mind (Alagöz et al., 2010) suggested a holistic approach for mobile e-health and wellness which reduces the healthcare cost using cloud computing environment. (Shimrat, 2009) define SWOT analysis for the role of cloud computing in healthcare and suggested that correctly implemented cloud computing infrastructure on local or hybrid cloud environment helps in providing better options for healthcare industries. HealthCloud (Doukas, Pliakas, & Maglogiannis, 2010) - a prototype, used commercially available cloud computing environment amazon S3 for storage of PHR and medical images using Android enabled mobile phone. Their implementation further needs security measures and user authentication on mobile phones. (Rolim et al., 2010) provided a solution based on integrating telemedicine services to automate the process from data collection to information delivery. This approach helps to collect data in real-time without any involvement of external factors that provide real-time data collection, eliminates the possibility of typing errors etc.

In Malaysia, the most of the hospitals process the information using computer-based information systems known as HIMS (Hospital Information & Management System) with the medical image processing software installed on the device that can review the MRI or X-Ray scan. (Ratnam & Dominic, 2012) suggested an infrastructure by pooling the resources from individual devices of HIMS to the single centralized cloud. The analysis of medical information requires huge processing power and large volumes of storage. Cloud computing based solutions helps to lower the operational cost. (Fan et al., 2011) presented a novel e-health approach based on DACAR (Data Capture and Auto Identification Reference). The DACAR platform provides authentication, authorization, secure data transmission, persistence, integrity, confidentiality and audit trail support for e-health. It also provides the suite of hardware and software solutions to integrate the capture, storage, and consumption of sensitive medical data along with large scale deployment and delivery of eHealths services using a cloud infrastructure.

Cloud-Sensor Infrastructure and Healthcare

A cloud can efficiently store a large amount of data and also process it efficiently. Though the wireless networks can sense the data, but they have limited processing power, small storage space, poor battery life and weak communication speeds. On the other hand, cloud computing offers high computation power, almost unlimited storage of structured as well as unstructured data, and above 99.99% uptime on high-speed communication links. The cloud resources are accessible from anywhere in the world using simple web-based interface, and the history of patient data can be reposited for the years on the cloud.

The wireless sensor networks play a vital role for the healthcare sector. There are hundreds of different diseases ranging from common cold to Parkinson's disease where cloud can be extensively used for securely access large amount of patient's data and made it available as when it required at different locations across the globe. The hybrid architecture of cloud and sensor networks as shown in Figure 4 is used in recent years to provide better infrastructure for the healthcare industry. They together efficiently monitor patients and provide services and analyze the patient's condition, report to doctors and attendants, facilitate them to provide better services to patients.

In the recent time, there are several researchers deployed cloud-sensor based architectures to provide services to healthcare sectors. Alamri et al. (2013)and Hossain and Muhammad (2014) presented the hybrid application and approaches to these two technologies and suggested a model for sensor-cloud based healthcare monitoring. Demiris, Hensel, Skubic, and Rantz (2008) tried to monitor body sugar, temperature and patients sleep condition by implementing wireless sensor devices. They used a mobile phone (GPRS), wi-fi gateway to transmit and store data to the cloud where they are processed further. Some researchers (Jit, Maniyeri, Louis, & Philip, 2009) designed a system which seamlessly support scale up and scale down of sensing devices i.e. they are highly adaptable towards the addition of newer sensor devices. In this system, after processing data at backend, the results are accessible through different devices like PDA, smart Phone or PC. The system

Figure 4. Sensor-based cloud infrastructures in healthcare monitoring

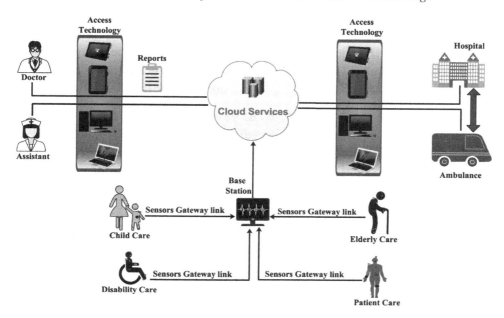

supports interactive web-based interface to fetch out and analyze the results (K. Lee, Murray, Hughes, & Joosen, 2010). With wearable body sensor network deployed over patient's body, there is one most common problem is a discontinuity of devices due to patients movement to perform their day-to-day routine activities. A system must be robust enough so that it supports multiple disconnections and also the data is not lost during the disconnection periods (Biswas, Jayachandran, Shue, Gopalakrishnan, & Yap, 2009).

CONCLUSION

The wireless networks are capable of sensing data in adverse conditions but they are limited by processing power, low storage space, battery life and communication speeds. On the other hand, cloud computing offers high computation power, almost unlimited storage of structured as well as unstructured data, 99.99% uptime and high-speed communication links. The cloud resources are accessible from anywhere in the world using simple web-based interface and the history of patient data can be kept for years on the cloud. A conflate framework of these two technologies may lead to a great architecture for future health monitoring systems making everywhere, everyone, anytime healthcare to be a reality.

REFERENCES

Abu-Faraj, Z. O., Akar, H. A., Assaf, E. H., Al-Qadiri, M. N., & Youssef, E. G. (2010). Evaluation of fall and fall recovery in a simulated seismic environment: A pilot study. In *Proceedings of the EEE Annual International Conference of the IEngineering in Medicine and Biology Society (EMBC'10)*. doi:10.1109/IEMBS.2010.5627696

Acampora, G., Cook, D. J., Rashidi, P., & Vasilakos, A. V. (2013). A survey on ambient intelligence in healthcare. *Proceedings of the IEEE, 101*(12), 2470–2494. doi:10.1109/JPROC.2013.2262913 PMID:24431472

Alagöz, F., Calero Valdez, A., Wilkowska, W., Ziefle, M., Dorner, S., & Holzinger, A. (2010). From cloud computing to mobile Internet, from user focus to culture and hedonism: The crucible of mobile health care and Wellness applications. In *Proceedings of 5th International Conference on Pervasive Computing and Applications (ICPCA'10)*. doi:10.1109/ICPCA.2010.5704072

Alamri, A., Ansari, W. S., Hassan, M. M., Hossain, M. S., Alelaiwi, A., & Hossain, M. A. (2013). A survey on sensor-cloud: Architecture, applications, and approaches. *International Journal of Distributed Sensor Networks, 2013*, 1–18. doi:10.1155/2013/917923

Alecsandru, R., Pruehsner, W., & Enderle, J. D. (1999). Remote Environmental Controller. In *Proceedings of the IEEE 25th Annual Northeast Bioengineering Conference*. IEEE.

Alemdar, H., & Ersoy, C. (2010). Wireless sensor networks for healthcare: A survey. *Computer Networks, 54*(15), 2688–2710. doi:10.1016/j.comnet.2010.05.003

Anderson, D., Luke, R. H., Keller, J. M., Skubic, M., Rantz, M., & Aud, M. (2009). Linguistic summarization of video for fall detection using voxel person and fuzzy logic. *Computer Vision and Image Understanding, 113*(1), 80–89. doi:10.1016/j.cviu.2008.07.006 PMID:20046216

Bagala, F., Becker, C., Cappello, A., Chiari, L., Aminian, K., Hausdorff, J. M., & Klenk, J. et al. (2012). Evaluation of accelerometer-based fall detection algorithms on real-world falls. *PLoS ONE, 7*(5), 1–9. doi:10.1371/journal.pone.0037062 PMID:22615890

Betke, M., Gips, J., & Fleming, P. (2002). The camera mouse: Visual tracking of body features to provide computer access for people with severe disabilities. *IEEE Transactions on Neural Systems and Rehabilitation Engineering, 10*(1), 1–10. doi:10.1109/TNSRE.2002.1021581 PMID:12173734

Bianchi, F., Redmond, S. J., Narayanan, M. R., Cerutti, S., & Lovell, N. H. (2010). Barometric pressure and triaxial accelerometry-based falls event detection. *IEEE Transactions on Neural Systems and Rehabilitation Engineering, 18*(6), 619–627. doi:10.1109/TNSRE.2010.2070807 PMID:20805056

Biswas, J., Jayachandran, M., Shue, L., Gopalakrishnan, K., & Yap, P. (2009). *Design and trial deployment of a practical sleep activity pattern monitoring system. In Ambient Assistive Health and Wellness Management in the Heart of the City* (pp. 190–200). Springer.

Bohonos, S., Lee, A., Malik, A., Thai, C., & Manduchi, R. (2007). Universal real-time navigational assistance (URNA): an urban bluetooth beacon for the blind. In *Proceedings of the 1st ACM international workshop on Systems and networking support for healthcare and assisted living environments (SIGMOBILE'07).* doi:10.1145/1248054.1248080

Bourke, A. K., O'Brien, J. V., & Lyons, G. M. (2007). Evaluation of a threshold-based tri-axial accelerometer fall detection algorithm. *Gait & Posture, 26*(2), 194–199. doi:10.1016/j.gaitpost.2006.09.012 PMID:17101272

Bourke, A. K., van de Ven, P., Gamble, M., O'Connor, R., Murphy, K., Bogan, E., & Nelson, J. et al. (2010). Assessment of waist-worn tri-axial accelerometer based fall-detection algorithms using continuous unsupervised activities. In *Proceedings of IEEE Annual International Conference of the Engineering in Medicine and Biology Society (EMBC'10).* doi:10.1109/IEMBS.2010.5626364

Chen, J., Kwong, K., Chang, D., Luk, J., & Bajcsy, R. (2006). Wearable sensors for reliable fall detection. In *Proceedings of the 27th Annual International Conference of the Engineering in Medicine and Biology Society* (IEEE-EMBS'05). doi:10.1109/IEMBS.2005.1617246

Chen, Y.-L. (2001). Application of tilt sensors in human-computer mouse interface for people with disabilities. *IEEE Transactions on Neural Systems and Rehabilitation Engineering, 9*(3), 289–294. doi:10.1109/7333.948457 PMID:11561665

Chuah, M., & DiBlasio, M. (2012). Smartphone based autism social alert system. In *Proceedings of the 8th International Conference on Mobile Ad-hoc and Sensor Networks (MSN'12).*

Coughlan, J., & Manduchi, R. (2007). Color targets: Fiducials to help visually impaired people find their way by camera phone. *EURASIP Journal on Image and Video Processing.*

Cucchiara, R., Prati, A., & Vezzani, R. (2007). A multi-camera vision system for fall detection and alarm generation. *Expert Systems: International Journal of Knowledge Engineering and Neural Networks, 24*(5), 334–345. doi:10.1111/j.1468-0394.2007.00438.x

Demiris, G., Hensel, B., Skubic, M., & Rantz, M. (2008). Senior residents' perceived need of and preferences for``smart home''sensor technologies. *International Journal of Technology Assessment in Health Care, 24*(1), 120–124. doi:10.1017/S0266462307080154 PMID:18218177

Diraco, G., Leone, A., & Siciliano, P. (2010). An active vision system for fall detection and posture recognition in elderly healthcare. In *Proceedings of the Design, Automation & Test in Europe Conference & Exhibition* (DATE'10).

Doukas, C., Pliakas, T., & Maglogiannis, I. (2010). Mobile healthcare information management utilizing Cloud Computing and Android OS. In *Proceedings of the IEEE Annual International Conference of the Engineering in Medicine and Biology Society (EMBC'10)*. IEEE.

El Alamy, L., Lhaddad, S., Maalal, S., Taybi, Y., & Salih-Alj, Y. (2012). Bus Identification System for Visually Impaired Person. In *Proceedings of the 6th International Conference on Next Generation Mobile Applications, Services and Technologies (NGMAST'12)*. doi:10.1109/NGMAST.2012.22

Fan, L., Buchanan, W., Thummler, C., Lo, O., Khedim, A., Uthmani, O., & Bell, D. et al. (2011). DACAR Platform for eHealth Services Cloud. In *Proceedings of the IEEE International Conference on Cloud Computing (CLOUD'11)*.

Fu, Z., Delbruck, T., Lichtsteiner, P., & Culurciello, E. (2008). An address-event fall detector for assisted living applications. *IEEE Transactions on Biomedical Circuits and Systems, 2*(2), 88–96. doi:10.1109/TBCAS.2008.924448 PMID:23852755

Ganz, A., Schafer, J., Gandhi, S., Puleo, E., Wilson, C., & Robertson, M. (2012). PERCEPT indoor navigation system for the blind and visually impaired: Architecture and experimentation. *International Journal of Telemedicine and Applications, 2012*, 19. doi:10.1155/2012/894869 PMID:23316225

Hazelhoff, L., & Han, J. (2008). Video-based fall detection in the home using principal component analysis. In *Proceedings of the Advanced Concepts for Intelligent Vision Systems*. doi:10.1007/978-3-540-88458-3_27

Helal, A., Moore, S. E., & Ramachandran, B. (2001). Drishti: An integrated navigation system for visually impaired and disabled. In *Proceedings of the 5th International Symposium on Wearable Computers*. doi:10.1109/ISWC.2001.962119

HIPPA. (1996). *Health Insurance Portability and Accountability Act of 1996 (HIPPA)*. Retrieved from: http://aspe.hhs.gov/admnsimp/p1104191.htm

Hossain, M. S., & Muhammad, G. (2014). Cloud-based collaborative media service framework for healthcare. *International Journal of Distributed Sensor Networks, 2014*, 1–11.

Igual, R., Medrano, C., & Plaza, I. (2013). Challenges, issues and trends in fall detection systems. *Biomedical Engineering Online, 12*(1), 66–66. doi:10.1186/1475-925X-12-66 PMID:23829390

Jit, B., Maniyeri, J., Louis, S., & Philip, Y. L. K. (2009). *Fast matching of sensor data with manual observations.* Paper presented at the Annual International Conference of the IEEE Engineering in Medicine and Biology Society. doi:10.1109/IEMBS.2009.5333881

Juan, C., Xiang, C., & Minfen, S. (2013). A framework for daily activity monitoring and fall detection based on surface electromyography and accelerometer signals. *IEEE Journal of Biomedical and Health Informatics, 17*(1), 38-45.

Kangas, M., Konttila, A., Lindgren, P., Winblad, I., & Timo, J. (2008). Comparison of low-complexity fall detection algorithms for body attached accelerometers. *Gait & Posture, 28*(2), 285–291. doi:10.1016/j.gaitpost.2008.01.003 PMID:18294851

Kangas, M., Vikman, I., Wiklander, J., Lindgren, P., Nyberg, L., & Timo, J. (2009). Sensitivity and specificity of fall detection in people aged 40 years and over. *Gait & Posture, 29*(4), 571–574. doi:10.1016/j.gaitpost.2008.12.008 PMID:19153043

Krasij, A. B., Pruehsner, W., & Enderle, J. D. (1999). VoxyBox. In *Proceedings of the 25th IEEE Annual Northeast Bioengineering Conference*. doi:10.1109/NEBC.1999.755767

Kupryjanow, A., Kunka, B., & Kostek, B. (2010). UPDRS Tests for Diagnosis of Parkinson's Disease Employing Virtual-Touchpad. In *Proceedings of the DEXA Workshops*. doi:10.1109/DEXA.2010.87

Lai, C.-F., Chang, S.-Y., Chao, H.-C., & Huang, Y.-M. (2011). Detection of cognitive injured body region using multiple tri-axial accelerometers for elderly falling. *IEEE Sensors Journal, 11*(3), 763–770. doi:10.1109/JSEN.2010.2062501

Lee, K., Murray, D., Hughes, D., & Joosen, W. (2010). *Extending sensor networks into the cloud using amazon web services.* Paper presented at the IEEE International Conference on Networked Embedded Systems for Enterprise Applications (NESEA 2010). doi:10.1109/NESEA.2010.5678063

Lee, T., & Mihailidis, A. (2005). An intelligent emergency response system: Preliminary development and testing of automated fall detection. *Journal of Telemedicine and Telecare, 11*(4), 194–198. doi:10.1258/1357633054068946 PMID:15969795

Lee, Y.-B., & Lee, M.-H. (2009). Indoor Positioning System for Moving Objects on an Indoor for Blind or Visually Impaired Playing Various Sports. *Proceedings of Journal of Electrical Engineering And Technology, 4*(1), 131–134. doi:10.5370/JEET.2009.4.1.131

LeMoyne, R., Coroian, C., & Mastroianni, T. (2009). Quantification of Parkinson's disease characteristics using wireless accelerometers. In *Proceedings of International Conference on Complex Medical Engineering (ICME'09)*. doi:10.1109/ICCME.2009.4906657

LeMoyne, R., Mastroianni, T., Cozza, M., Coroian, C., & Grundfest, W. (2010). Implementation of an iPhone for characterizing Parkinson's disease tremor through a wireless accelerometer application. In *Proceedings of IEEE Annual International Conference of the Engineering in Medicine and Biology Society (EMBC'10)*. doi:10.1109/IEMBS.2010.5627240

Li, M., Yu, S., Ren, K., & Lou, W. (2010). *Securing personal health records in cloud computing: Patient-centric and fine-grained data access control in multi-owner settings. In Security and Privacy in Communication Networks* (pp. 89–106). Springer.

Li, Q., Stankovic, J. A., Hanson, M. A., Barth, A. T., Lach, J., & Zhou, G. (2009). Accurate, fast fall detection using gyroscopes and accelerometer-derived posture information. In *Proceedings of 6th International Workshop on Wearable and Implantable Body Sensor Networks (BSN'09)*. doi:10.1109/BSN.2009.46

Libelium. (2015). *50 Sensor Applications for a Smarter World*. Author.

Lin, C.-W., & Ling, Z.-H. (2007). Automatic fall incident detection in compressed video for intelligent homecare. In *Proceedings of the 16th International Conference on Computer Communications and Networks (ICCCN'07)*. doi:10.1109/ICCCN.2007.4317978

Lin, Q., Zhang, D., Ni, H., Zhou, X., & Yu, Z. (2012). An Integrated Service Platform for Pervasive Elderly Care. In *Proceedings of the IEEE Asia-Pacific Services Computing Conference (APSCC'12)*. doi:10.1109/APSCC.2012.21

Lindemann, U., Hock, A., Stuber, M., Keck, W., & Becker, C. (2005). Evaluation of a fall detector based on accelerometers: A pilot study. *Medical & Biological Engineering & Computing, 43*(5), 548–551. doi:10.1007/BF02351026 PMID:16411625

Liu, C.-L., Lee, C.-H., & Lin, P.-M. (2010). A fall detection system using k-nearest neighbor classifier. *Expert Systems with Applications*, *37*(10), 7174–7181. doi:10.1016/j.eswa.2010.04.014

McCann, J., Wang, H., Zheng, H., & Eccleston, C. (2012). An interactive assessment system for children with chronic pain. In *Proceedings of the IEEE-EMBS International Conference on Biomedical and Health Informatics (BHI'12)*. doi:10.1109/BHI.2012.6211739

Mell, P., & Grance, T. (2011). *The NIST definition of cloud computing*. Retrieved from:http://csrc.nist.gov/publications/nistpubs/800-145/SP800-145.pdf

Microsoft. (2015). *Health vault*. Microsoft Healthvault. available: https://www.healthvault.com/in/en

Ming, L., Shucheng, Y., Yao, Z., Kui, R., & Wenjing, L. (2012). Scalable and Secure Sharing of Personal Health Records in Cloud Computing Using Attribute-Based Encryption. *IEEE Transactions on Parallel and Distributed Systems*, *24*(1), 131–143. doi:10.1109/tpds.2012.97

Morrison, L. J. (1997). Major Incident Medical Management and Support: The Practical Approach. *CMAJ: Canadian Medical Association Journal*, *156*(1), 78.

Okuno, R., Yokoe, M., Fukawa, K., Sakoda, S., & Akazawa, K. (2007). Measurement system of finger-tapping contact force for quantitative diagnosis of Parkinson's disease. In *Proceedings of the 29th IEEE Annual International Conference of the Engineering in Medicine and Biology Society (EMBS'07)*. doi:10.1109/IEMBS.2007.4352549

Orwat, C., Graefe, A., & Faulwasser, T. (2008). Towards pervasive computing in health care-A literature review. *BMC Medical Informatics and Decision Making*, *8*(1), 26. doi:10.1186/1472-6947-8-26 PMID:18565221

Pantelopoulos, A., & Bourbakis, N. G. (2010). A survey on wearable sensor-based systems for health monitoring and prognosis. *IEEE Transactions on Systems, Man and Cybernetics. Part C, Applications and Reviews*, *40*(1), 1–12. doi:10.1109/TSMCC.2009.2032660

Pruette, C. S., Fadrowski, J. J., Bedra, M., & Finkelstein, J. (2013). Feasibility of a mobile blood pressure telemanagement system in children with hypertension. In *Proceedings of the IEEE Point-of-Care Healthcare Technologies (PHT'13)*. doi:10.1109/PHT.2013.6461316

Rakocevic, G. (2009). Overview of sensors for wireless sensor networks. *Transactions on Internet Research*, *5*, 13–18.

Ran, L., Helal, S., & Moore, S. (2004). Drishti: an integrated indoor/outdoor blind navigation system and service. In *Proceedings of the 2nd IEEE Annual Conference on Pervasive Computing and Communications (PerCom'04)* doi:10.1109/PERCOM.2004.1276842

Ratnam, K. A., & Dominic, P. D. D. (2012). Cloud services - Enhancing the Malaysian healthcare sector. In *Proceedings of the International Conference on Computer & Information Science (ICCIS'12)*.

Rimminen, H., Lindström, J., Linnavuo, M., & Sepponen, R. (2010). Detection of falls among the elderly by a floor sensor using the electric near field. *IEEE Transactions on Information Technology in Biomedicine, 14*(6), 1475-1476.

Rolim, C. O., Koch, F. L., Westphall, C. B., Werner, J., Fracalossi, A., & Salvador, G. S. (2010). A Cloud Computing Solution for Patient's Data Collection in Health Care Institutions. In *Proceedings of the Second International Conference on eHealth, Telemedicine, and Social Medicine* (ETELEMED '10).

Shaou-Gang, M., Pei-Hsu, S., & Chia-Yuan, H. (2006). A Customized Human Fall Detection System Using Omni-Camera Images and Personal Information. In *Proceedings of the 1st Transdisciplinary Conference on Distributed Diagnosis and Home Healthcare* (D2H2'06).

Shima, K., Tamura, Y., Tsuji, T., Kandori, A., Yokoe, M., & Sakoda, S. (2008). Estimation of human finger tapping forces based on a fingerpad-stiffness model. In *Proceedings of the IEEE Annual International Conference of the Engineering in Medicine and Biology Society (EMBC'09)*.

Shima, K., Tsuji, T., Kandori, A., Yokoe, M., & Sakoda, S. (2009). Measurement and evaluation of finger tapping movements using log-linearized Gaussian mixture networks. *Sensors (Basel, Switzerland), 9*(3), 2187–2201. doi:10.3390/s90302187 PMID:22574008

Shimrat, O. (2009). Cloud computing and healthcare. *San Diego Physician. Org*, 26-29.

Shucheng, Y., Cong, W., Kui, R., & Wenjing, L. (2010). Achieving Secure, Scalable, and Fine-grained Data Access Control in Cloud Computing. In *Proceedings of the IEEE INFOCOM*.

Starida, K., Ganiatsas, G., Fotiadis, D. I., & Likas, A. (2003). CHILDCARE: a collaborative environment for the monitoring of children healthcare at home. In *Proceedings of the 4th International IEEE EMBS Special Topic Conference on Information Technology Applications in Biomedicine*. doi:10.1109/ITAB.2003.1222501

Struijk, L. N. S. A. (2006). An inductive tongue computer interface for control of computers and assistive devices. *IEEE Transactions on Bio-Medical Engineering*, *53*(12), 2594–2597. doi:10.1109/TBME.2006.880871 PMID:17152438

Sultan, N. (2013). Making use of cloud computing for healthcare provision: Opportunities and challenges. *International Journal of Information Management*, *34*(2), 177–184. doi:10.1016/j.ijinfomgt.2013.12.011

Super, G., Groth, S., & Hook, R. (1994). *START: simple triage and rapid treatment plan*. Newport Beach, CA: Hoag Memorial Presbyterian Hospital.

Takami, O., Irie, N., Kang, C., Ishimatsu, T., & Ochiai, T. (1996). Computer interface to use head movement for handicapped people. In *Proceedings of the IEEE TENCON on Digital Signal Processing Applications (TENCON'96)*. doi:10.1109/TENCON.1996.608861

Takami, O., Morimoto, K., Ochiai, T., & Ishimatsu, T. (1995). Computer interface to use head and eyeball movement for handicapped people. In *Proceedings of the IEEE International Conference on Intelligent Systems for the 21st Century, Systems, Man and Cybernetics*. doi:10.1109/ICSMC.1995.537920

Tartamella, S. S., Pruehsner, W., & Enderle, J. D. (1999). Remote control digital thermostat and remote door opener. In *Proceedings of the IEEE 25ᵗʰ Annual Northeast Bioengineering Conference*. doi:10.1109/NEBC.1999.755759

Uniyal, D., & Raychoudhury, V. (2014). *Pervasive Healthcare-A Comprehensive Survey of Tools and Techniques*. arXiv preprint arXiv:1411.1821

Varshney, U. (2007). Pervasive healthcare and wireless health monitoring. *Mobile Networks and Applications*, *12*(2-3), 113–127. doi:10.1007/s11036-007-0017-1

Vishwakarma, V., Mandal, C., & Sural, S. (2007). *Automatic detection of human fall in video. In Pattern Recognition and Machine Intelligence* (pp. 616–623). Springer. doi:10.1007/978-3-540-77046-6_76

Visintin, M., Barbeau, H., Korner-Bitensky, N., & Mayo, N. E. (1998). A new approach to retrain gait in stroke patients through body weight support and treadmill stimulation. *Stroke*, *29*(6), 1122–1128. doi:10.1161/01.STR.29.6.1122 PMID:9626282

WHO. (2007). *Global report on falls prevention in older age*. World Health Organization.

WHO. (2015a). *The 10 leading causes of death in the world, 2000 and 2012*. Retrieved from http://www.who.int/mediacentre/factsheets/fs310/en/

WHO. (2015b). World Health Organization.

Williams, A., Ganesan, D., & Hanson, A. (2007). Aging in place: fall detection and localization in a distributed smart camera network. In *Proceedings of the 15th International Conference on Multimedia*. doi:10.1145/1291233.1291435

Wood, A., Stankovic, J. A., Virone, G., Selavo, L., He, Z., Cao, Q., & Stoleru, R. et al. (2008). Context-aware wireless sensor networks for assisted living and residential monitoring. *IEEE Network*, *22*(4), 26–33. doi:10.1109/MNET.2008.4579768

Yu, K.-H., Yoon, M.-J., & Jeong, G.-Y. (2013). Recognition of obstacle distribution via vibrotactile stimulation for the visually disabled. In *Proceedings of the IEEE International Conference on Mechatronics (ICM'13)*

Zhang, C., Tian, Y., & Capezuti, E. (2012). *Privacy preserving automatic fall detection for elderly using RGBD cameras*. Springer. doi:10.1007/978-3-642-31522-0_95

Chapter 3
Cloud Based Secure Data Sharing Algorithm for Health Care

Saravana Kumar N.
VIT University, India

Rajya Lakshmi Gubburi Venkataramana
Northwestern Polytechnic University, USA

Balamurugan B.
VIT University, India

ABSTRACT

Cloud computing is one of most fast developing technology and many organizations are now offering a wide range of cloud services. Although the services provided are the same there is no common programming language, technology and protocol to access the entirety of the cloud services. Client who use a service provided by a certain organization are often limited and confined to that specific organization its structure and technologies. A Cloud federation is one solution to that interoperability through which computing resources of one Cloud Service Provider is rented or sold to another service provider or the services provided by one Cloud Service Provider is replicated into another Cloud Service Provider without having to lose any functionality and performance. This process is a tedious task and is prone to multiple limitations. In this paper we proposed the architectural framework and algorithm for the possible interoperability between the cloud service providers based on SLA in prospective of health sector as the application of cloud in health sector is highly needed in future.

DOI: 10.4018/978-1-5225-1002-4.ch003

INTRODUCTION

The Cloud computing generally is a type of computing that relies upon sharing of computing resources rather than having the local servers or personal devices to handle application or services. Cloud computing may be defined as services accessed by means of Internet. The buzzword cloud transforms the way of storing and accessing the data. Unlike traditional applications the cloud applications are web specific in nature. To access cloud applications one needs to have the web supported device. Thus the cloud applications are platform independent and it can be accessed any time anywhere and any place. The ultimate aim of the cloud computing is to give everything as a service to the customers. In cloud computing generally there are three man services, SaaS (Software as a service), PaaS (Platform as a service) and IaaS the Infrastructure as service respectively. And it consists of three main deployment models public cloud, private and Hybrid cloud. In software as service, the software is being stored in cloud servers and it will be being accessed by the client and charges are being paid by the customer as per usage. The customer need not to install the software at the client end. There are several benefits both for client and the vendors. The client need not to have any knowledge of installation, processor speed, and memory in the host system as the service is being retrieved from the cloud servers. Most importantly the client is being charged as per use. In case of vendors, the usage of pirated software is reduced significantly. The Microsoft is planned to offer its software's everything through cloud. Thus software as a service require minimal amount knowledge to access various services. Whereas the Platform as a service is meant for the developers. It supports the various software development kit and automated testing environment. The infrastructure as a service generally meant for providing the services like hardware and memory support. There are many other services are available including storage as a service e.g. Drop box, security as service, monitoring as service, communication as a service etc. As discussed earlier, the cloud provides every needs of the customers as a service. Coming to deployment models, the public clouds is accessible anyone provided the access credentials and data center nearby the location. The public cloud is considered to be insecure and easily hacked. The private cloud is considered to be highly secure and data can be accessed within the organization environment and maintained by the either the cloud service provider or the local member of organization. The hybrid cloud generally the combination of any two cloud services.

The cloud services are considered to be hit. According to Gartner the revenue of the cloud has been increased gradually. The revenue of cloud computing in 2009 is about 58 billion US dollars where as in 2010 it is nearly 70 billion US dollars. There is 16-17 percent increase in revenue for academic year 2011. The cloud revenue in 2012 is about 111 billion US dollars and in 2013 it's about 130 US dollars. The cloud revenue is increasing day by day as every domain is started moving to cloud to utilize the characteristics and advantages of cloud. The various advantages include availability, cost, multi tenancy, security, maintainability, auditing etc. The reason behind the adaptation of cloud is its benefits (Figure 1). Unfortunately, its benefits are turned out to be its limitations. The major limitation of cloud is security. And there is tradeoff between the security, privacy and cost. The question arises who is responsible for protecting the data of the users. Though there are many encryption algorithm and better auditing techniques still cloud lack something behind. The cloud is secure but not cent percent. The important thing need to be addressed to improve the security, scalability and energy efficient computing is to make cloud interoperable cloud through federation.

At present cloud services are being offered in critical application domain like Health care diagnosis and in financial services. Unlike, early 20th century the customers are preferring cloud based services. Fear to adopt cloud services are being reduced. The diagram depicts the statement. Nowadays research in cloud are much concentrated on Inter-operable cloud services (Multi-cloud architectures), and energy efficient resource management. This is achieved by means of using Cloud-Federation. This makes cloud services providers for energy efficient routing and providing better services to the customers. Conflict is being raised here. No one is offering services for the end-users as the companies are concentrating much on their own revenues. This is the major reason for lot of research are being carried over in cloud federation and autonomic computing.

The health care plays vital role in every human being. The size of medical data like medical imaging, scan results are increasing exponentially for patient. The emergent of connected health is highly engaging for efficient sharing of data across

Figure 1. Revenue of cloud in billions

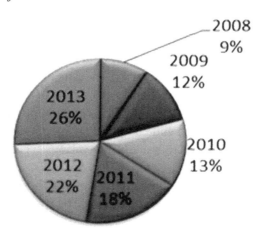

organization. The diagnosis of the patient will be based on the medication the patient had taken in the past which indeed helps the medical practitioners for identification of similar disease which affects the patients. As a result, it is advisable to maintain the single account for Personal Health Record (PHR) for the patient. And all the electronic Health record (EHR) of the patient are being stored in PHR. And the PHR are stored and maintained in the cloud service provider. The CSP needs to maintain high level data security and privacy of the data needs to be preserved. There is a rapid progress in medical field in terms of disease and treatment but still the storage of data and sharing of data is difficult. Data size of the health sector is very large and even single genome needs a lot of storage space. This leads to future research in health sector. Besides it needs high level data security and authentication with verifiable data availability. As a result, we have proposed the framework for health system for storing and accessing the medical data using cloud.

Background

The paper Ubiquitous Healthcare Services with a Novel Efficient Cloud Platform illustrates the need of accessing and sharing of health care data. The author proposes the framework for efficient data sharing using cloud. The paper is patient centric and author haven't described about the data management by the hospital or cloud service providers. Moreover, as per the guidelines of HIPAA it is not advisable to store the data in the public cloud as it is openly available in internet and it has high risk of getting hacked.

The article "efficient framework for health system based on hybrid cloud with ABE-outsourced decryption" describes the way for data storage and efficient sharing of data by means of using community cloud. As a result, the data sharing is limited to "N" number of Hospitals and it doesn't reduce cost of building infrastructure compared to traditional servers. Thus the framework fails in terms of cost by concentrating much on security and privacy of the data.

In order to overcome the issue, the article proposes Layered storage architecture for health system using cloud. The paper generally dealt with efficient storage of large amount of data based on the criticality of the data involved. The classification of data is done based on type of medication and stored in either private, public or hybrid cloud. The framework uses Attribute based encryption techniques along with RC5 algorithm for Access control and encryption respectively. Though it seems to be promising it's highly difficult to manage the various types of data and it need to be synchronized.

The paper" cloud cluster communication accessing C-MPICH for critical application overcomes the above described problem. The concept of message passing interface have been introduced and thus secure communication between the system and the server being connected can be carried over. The clouds server is being clustered. Albeit, the system seems to be efficient the accessing of data are limited to particular cluster. As the authentication of system were carried over using the IP address, the storage and access control are denied to the particular cluster. Thus the framework is highly scalable indeed it's not ubiquitous.

The cloud Inter-connected cloud computing Environments: challenges, Taxonomy and survey illustrates the need of cloud federation and inter-cloud communication. The author describes the various issues involves in the inter-cloud communication and ways to overcome. The Service level agreements plays a vital in it. The paper "common cloud architecture for cloud Interoperability overcomes the all the limitation of the existing system and describes framework for efficient data transfer in the cloud. The paper doesn't concentrate on storage of data and access control techniques indeed it provides efficient framework for inter-cloud connectivity. The article "Enhanced attribute based encryption for cloud computing" portrays the need of different encryption algorithm based on the criticality of the data involved in the cloud. The article classifies the applications based on some factors with suitable encryption algorithm. Finally proposed the light-weight Attribute based encryption for the critical application for cloud computing like health care.

An Efficient Framework and access control scheme for cloud health care portrays the importance of security in data sharing using the concept of Inter-operability of cloud services. Moreover, the paper also describes about algorithm for the data sharing in cloud using outsourced Decryption concentrating much in decryption of the data. The algorithm is the extension of the Verifiable Outsourced Decryption scheme proposed by Lai. The implementation was carried over using charm crypto system which is the statistical open source tool for algorithm validation.

NEED IMPORTANCE OF CLOUD FEDERATION

The background shows the brief idea that cloud based health care is hot research area. Our framework is based on the public cloud scenario it reduces cost of the data sharing but it not publicly available to anyone who accessing the services. As the medical need to maintain the privacy and security and need to have less maintenance cost it is advisable to move to cloud federation. Every data transfer is monitored by the autonomic cloud. Generally, cloud federation is nothing but the transfer of data by maintaining common SLA between the two or more service providers. Firstly, we see the importance of cloud federation.

Vendor Locking

The one of the most important thing is vendor locking. The customer is being locked to certain vendors for its services. There will be detailed Service level agreements between the vendors and customers. But there are certain cases where the SLA fails. Some XYZ Company registered for cloud service to "K" vendor. Suddenly vendor decided not to offer cloud services to any client or client. Client cannot able to move to other vendor as it has different architecture and storage techniques. If the client need to shift to another vendor the client needs to pay huge amount to shift to new vendor. It is difficult to move to other vendor in future as cloud doesn't have any proper standardization like traditional networking. Every cloud vendor has its own architecture and it is less transparent. Thus client should not depend upon the service provider for any cause. Thus cloud federation is much needed to overcome the risk of vendor locking

Resource Allocation

The term federation generally defined is common understanding between the two cloud service providers. If two or more similar data being stored in different cloud providers is waste of storage and energy. By means of using cloud federation the effective resource is being utilized and the virtual images are being transferred from the one cloud service similar kind of data that can be shared between the two campuses by federation through common understanding between the vendors. Thus provides the effective resource utilization and scalability between two campuses for a particular locality. Data can be even transferred to any other partner universities across the globe by means of federation.

Distribution Across Clouds

Some vendors may not have their infrastructure in some geographical locations. By means of federation this limitation is overcome. Thus service can be provided to any customer where it has no infrastructure. This indeed results in cost effective approach. Thus data is being spread across the clouds. These where the three important reasons why cloud federation is needed. Every company moves towards cloud federation and Inter-operability. Specifically, CISCO is moving from private cloud to Inter-cloud communication. Cisco is not offered any public cloud services to the end user like amazon or Microsoft. The CISCO is much concentrated providing services to the companies or organization. CISCO is spent nearly 2 billion dollars to make inter-cloud feasible by maintaining SLA with nearly 40 cloud vendors in different geographical location. The CISCO uses its own fabric to connect the various vendors. Thus enabling secure transformation of data across the multiple clouds.

CHALLENGES INVOLVED IN CLOUD FEDERATION

Identification of Clouds

The cloud identification is one of the challenges involved. The resource needs to transfer to the appropriate cloud which is being requested. This course of action (request and response) takes place by means of brokering services using middleware. The clouds are identified semantically. The broker service should be autonomic in nature.

VM Migration

Once the clouds are being identified the virtual machine image need to migrate from one cloud to another. This again a difficult task. Currently for VM migration there are many concepts and tools. VMotion and XEN are the live migration techniques proposed by the VM Ware and Intel respectively. The many things are considered in VM live migration like down time, replication time, memory etc. VM migration needs to be done from one cloud to another.

Service Level Agreements

The service level agreements need to maintain between the cloud providers and the end users. The SLA plays a vital role in the Inter-operability of clouds. Without SLA between the cloud providers the inter-operability by means of federation is not feasible. Thus the cloud service provider must agree to for the federation.

Load Balancing

The load balancing technique need to follow in cloud especially in cloud federation as the cloud VM are being migrated from the one cloud to another. The user request and memory are need to manage. Usually the hardware is used for the load balancing but it increases the cost of the system. Currently software defined networks are being used in place of hardware and switch. This helps in auto scaling of the cloud servers. But the drawback of software defined networks is its performance degradation compare to the software defined networks. The HAVEN (Holistic load balancing and auto scaling approach) provides solution to the performance problem.

Legal Issues and Standardization

There are many legal issue in connecting the cloud. Since cloud has many outages it needs to follow and abide the rules before connecting it. In US there are many agencies like FBI has the rights to check the data in public cloud without permission from the service providers. That's the main reason why the CISCO is moving towards the inter-connected private clouds rather than public clouds. HIPPA act to prevent storing the health data in public cloud. The European and Asian countries have own legal issues. The each and every cloud has its own storage, encryption and access techniques and varies from service providers. The NIST cloud computing Inter-operability standards to be followed. The ultimate aim is to transfer the VM images from the one cloud to another.

Security and Confidentiality

The cloud architecture is not transparent like Traditional Network architecture. For interoperability the common standard architecture needs to be followed. The transparent architecture will increase the confidence to the users. The IEEE is initiated the towards the common reference architecture for the cloud inter-operability. The secure transfer of data from cloud need to takes place. The security and privacy are the major concerns that ultimately depends upon the cloud architecture and models. Thus the end users' needs to trust the cloud service provider. The insider attack needs to be overcome. Thus the main reason for moving towards the autonomic cloud. The data confidentiality needs to achieve as the data is outsourced from one cloud to another. The data should not be modifying which is sent thus verifiable outsource of data need to be done while transferring the VM images.

Monitoring and Access Policies

There are various methods available to monitor the cloud services. The strength and weakness of the cloud need to monitor 24/7. The amount of data being sent and acknowledgement of the data are to be done by the monitoring tool. In case of any significant changes the process need to turn off by themselves. The access policy plays a vital role in inter-operability of cloud. The access policy should be ontology or semantically connected virtual networks and the broker service has the knowledge of the various clouds. If the access policy fails, the cloud interoperability fails and may lead to data leakage to some unauthorized users/cloud.

Auditing

The auditing refers to overall monitoriztion of the service whether the any deviation from the proposed architecture. The auditing involves not only the data transfer. It also involves the whole communication process. Third party auditing is to be done by the consortium. There is a chance third party and Cloud Service Provider will collude with each other. Therefore, the random auditing to be done by the cloud service provider to the middleware intelligent cloud. Our architecture uses using algebraic signatures to check data possession in cloud storage. In case of Inter-cloud communication, the major thing to be audit the security. Every cloud need to communicate with each other without affecting the privacy of the users involved in it. Especially data leakage where access control plays a vital role. Since we have mentioned autonomic cloud, there is no user intervention thus results no a point of insider attack. May be the deviation is caused by threat, or malicious attack by the hackers. Various hindrances may occur for cloud data owner to keep its data intact and available on the cloud. The problems can be because of ignorance of cloud service providers, the cloud data provider's agreement with auditor to hide their mistakes, cloud auditor mishandling and improper auditing. These problems are major threats for data and application owner as well its users which results in loss of data integrity and leads to in-appropriation of results consequently leads to major loses (financial loss or loss of life). To prevent these kinds of major loses especially in case of critical applications; we propose a method to randomly double check data integrity and availability over cloud (Figure 2). This method is enhancement of available TPAs where (1) Standard ISO/IEC 27007 which has specific guidelines to ensure proper auditing is deployed and (2) A self-audit mechanism for data owner to ensure data integrity and availability on cloud and match it with results provided by the TPAs.

C: → DO*TPA

where the communication between the Data owner and Third Party Auditor. The scheme to double check is a random audit validation. In this the Data Owner provides a periodic audit challenge to the TPAs. The TPA in return completes the specified audits and presents the results $\{A_1, A_2, ..., A_n\}$ to the Data Owner. The results set $\{A_1, A_2, ..., A_n\}$ becomes the sample space. Then, the Data Owner checks the audit reports and makes a match with given challenge, which assures the TPA's has completed challenge. But to assure that the given challenge has been completed as expected.

Figure 2. Proposed self-auditing system

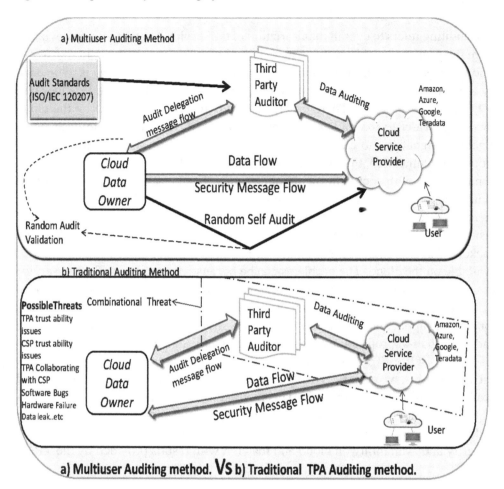

a) Multiuser Auditing method. **Vs** b) Traditional TPA Auditing method.

PROPOSED WORK

We have proposed various hypothesis related to cloud federation and cloud interoperability for health care.

H1: Transparency of Cloud Might Leads to Theft

One the most controversial belief is that federation of cloud requires the CSP to reveal its underlying architecture to facilitate interoperability and this will increase the amount of attacks on the CSP. This is not entirely true since a security feature should not depend on the attacker's ignorance but rather it should be on the integrity of the architecture to withstand such attacks. Most of the network architecture is transparent but do not face as many attacks due to their integrity. Most of the problems mainly caused by known reasons rather than unknown reasons this is a result of lack of diligence in creating a secure health cloud. And thus a standard secure architecture is much needed for interoperability.

H2: Can it Be Developed by Single Organization?

The answer is obviously no. The company needs to have much investment but still not possible. The single organization cannot be maintained and provide all the services to the client. Thus to promote inter-operability and cloud federation there should be mutual agreement between the company. Even the amazon the largest web service provider not able to provider all the services to the customer. And maintenance is too difficult. Thus inter-operability is much needed with common goal and SLA.

H3: Cloud Federation is Achieved Across the Globe Among CSP

Can the federation globally integrate every CSP there is, probably not. Each company likes to increase their own revenue and promote themselves. Some of the major Cloud Service Providers such as Amazon, Microsoft, IBM, Infosys, Google, etc. are interested towards a common cloud architecture but they cannot force organizations such as CISCO which prefer an inter-related network of private clouds as they prefer privacy over interoperability. They are not at fault here and it is their right to choose their own policy but this prevents a globalization of the federation. The most common reason is distrust among CSP's as well as competition among them.

CLOUD FEDERATION FRAMEWORK

There are various clouds computing services and data centers in different geographical locations around the world. The conceptual diagram of cloud federation across the globe is given in Figure 3.

We have proposed the framework for cloud federation. All the clouds are being connected semantically. All clouds are semantically connected to each other based on the attributes involved using domain. For example, the medical domain, all the attributes are connected to each other. Every cloud has its own data storage and encryption technique therefore one cannot simply transfer the source or data from one cloud to other. This actually needs the proper authorization before implementing the strategy. The autonomic cloud (middleware) takes care the authorization

Figure 3. Basic architectural overview: Cloud federation

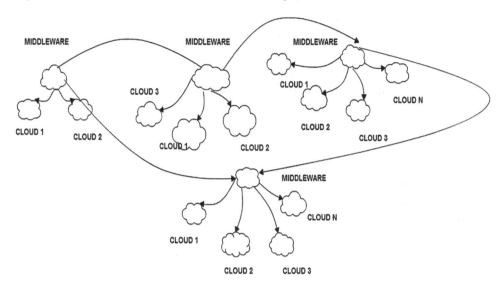

techniques my means of semantic interoperability. Indeed, needs to maintain common Service level agreements as it involves multiple CSPs. In our proposed system we are using the Ontology based semantic connectivity between the clouds.

Algorithm

Step 1: Let A_1, A_2...n $\in$ C are clouds.
Step 2: Let p_1, p_2, p_3.....p_n $\in$ P (Users)
For $P_i \in P$, $P \in C$. I.e. every user belongs to any one of the cloud service provider.
$\forall C \exists A$, where A- Autonomic cloud (Responsible for cloud federation), provided SLA

Instance

When a user makes a request, the request is being transferred to autonomic cloud. Using Meta data, the cloud chooses the CSP and provide access back to the client.

User (Pi) $\xrightarrow{request}$ Service to C. (usually by means of XACML)

C $\xrightarrow{request}$ A (Autonomic cloud)

A $\xrightarrow{Meta\ data}$ chooses CSP.

The CSP are chooses among the various providers based on request. The client may either need the service, or just the processer for processing the data. This is done using the RDF.

In case of data,

$$A \xrightarrow{\text{responses}} C \ (Pi) \text{ with VM images.}$$

The VM images are again transferred into common data format XACML/XML for human read. At last, Acknowledgement needs to provide to the autonomic cloud. And whole process needs to be monitored by standard organization. Basically, the performance will be slower compared to the normal cloud service provider though the processing power increases drastically. As it takes time to identify the cloud service and response it back. Everything needs to be standardized in cloud federation before implementing it. Moreover, the accuracy of data being received or cloud services being opted is ultimately depends upon the factor of semantic cloud. This act as a backbone for the cloud interoperability. Attribute based encryption with outsourced decryption provides better solution with verifiability of data. The more transparent architecture indeed responsible for the large outages and attacks in Virtual server. Thus there is always tradeoff between transparency and security. By means of cloud federation vendor locking is avoided, increased performance and secure transfer of data from one cloud to another.

The clouds are semantically connected using ontology. The term "ontology referred to degree of relationship between the two or more objects. Here the degree of relationship between the two or more clouds are calculated and semantically being connected. If the service is needed by the end user /customer, then it searches the data or service available in the particular location based nearer to the server. And if the requested service is unavailable then it requests the middleware of the nearby virtual server and it passes through the checks by using the Meta data available. Finally, the requested data are transferred to the client. The clouds are being connected using the geographical location and with respect to the domain. This is the basic pre-requisite. Figure 4 represents the detailed diagram how the cloud federation are being implemented. Figure 5 is the pseudo code for the proposed algorithm.

System Design

The System design consist of the following automation phases and it is represented as CF.

CF= {M, C, F, R, O, T}, Where CF is quantified.

Figure 4. Detailed diagram representing cloud federation

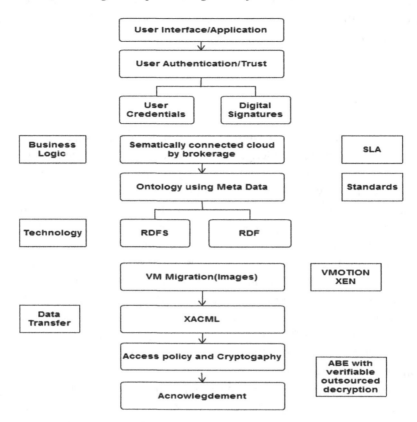

Figure 5. Pseudo code of proposed Algorithm

Algorithm 1 CLOUD FEDERATION

article algorithmic

1: **procedure** SERVICE REQUEST (▷)by customer
2:     Ci of $Pi \leftarrow request$
3:     **while** $Si \neq CSP$ **do**
4:         $Mi \leftarrow Ci$
5:         **return** $Service$
        $Si \leftarrow Mi$
6:         **while** $Si = Mi$ **do**
    $ci \leftarrow Mi$
7:             **return** $Service$
    else

8:             **return** $Service Not Found$
9:

1. M, is the set of Middleware's associated with that." M_t is defined as Middleware which is being transferred at time "t". Let m_1.....m_n be set of Middleware that were spread across geographically based on semantic ontology.

$$M = \{m_1, m_2, m_3 \ldots\ldots m_n\}$$

2. "C" is the set of clouds associated with the "M". $C \in M$

$$C = \{C_1, C_2, C_3 \ldots.. C_n\}$$

3. "F" is the set of functions associated with the Cloud customers "C" and the it is Input to the automatic cloud at the instance of "t"

$$F = \{f_1, f_2, f_3 \ldots\ldots f_n\}$$

4. "R" is the set of responses associated with the Function "f" at the instance of time "t" and R is the output of the autonomic cloud.

$$R = \{r_1, r_2, r_3 \ldots.. r_n\}$$

5. "O" is the set of attributes associated with the clouds. The attributes are semantically connected across the clouds

$$O = \{o_1, o_2, o_3 \ldots\ldots o_n\}$$

6. "T" is the operation and it denotes the degree of relationship between the Functions associated with cloud and the ontological attribute with the other cloud which is governed by the Middleware.

$$T = \{F \times O\}$$

The framework portrays how the data are being transferred from one CSP to another and to the user. The data are being encrypted using ABE and one authorization to the client by means of satisfying the access structure the patient can transfer the data to the person. The data are usually transferred by XACML format.

Scheduling Algorithm

1. Each middleware consist of cloud service being associated with that.

$M_1 = \{C_1, C_2, C_3, \dots C_n\}$

2. Probability of selecting the event that are mutually exclusive will depends upon

$P(fi) = (P(C_1), P(C_2)\dots\dots\dots P(C_n))$

3. The probability of system reliability is calculated by using

$$\text{Reliability} = \prod_{i=1}^{n} Fi$$

The selecting the cloud service follows the Greedy algorithm for optimal solution required by the "service".

Though the greedy algorithm never gives optimal solution to the problem associated as it searches the query based on heuristic. Moreover, Greedy algorithm looks after all the nodes associated with it. Thus in turn gives the optimal solution for the case of the problem. Finally, the requested service or processor or anything is transferred to the customer. The greedy algorithm is efficient for combinatorial problems.

Once the appropriate Middleware is selected, the Algorithm follows Bayer's' rule, where the Probability of occurring event is classified into two or more types.

For example, the probability of occurring the event "A" is classified into the two or more clouds. We are describing the clouds as events.

$$P(A) = \sum_{f=i}^{n} P\left(\frac{f}{Mi}\right), P(Mi)$$

where the probability of occurring the event is totally based on the middleware.

$$P(A) = \sum_{f=i}^{n} P\left(\frac{Mi}{Ci}\right), P(Ci)$$

Once the middleware is being selected the probability of event is based on the cloud service providers.

DISCUSSION AND IMPLEMENTATION SOLUTION

The cloud federation is the hot topic in cloud computing. The implementation and maintenance of the cloud federation in large scale across the globe is difficult. By means of using cloud federation, the user data are easily transferred to different hospitals across the globe for effective treatment to the patient. The patient can easily share the data with various friends and relatives and to insurance companies to remove frauds. The patient can access the medical records, the data of visit to hospital, and the medicine prescribed by the hospital for treatment can be viewed easily using any devices that are capable of connecting to internet. This indeed reduces the cost of treatment and effective sharing of the EHR has been made. The data analytics plays a vital role. With the help of Meta data, it is easy for the researches to find out the person affected from certain diseases and it easier to treat and discover medicines based on heuristic data. Moreover, it is easier for the patient to keep track the medicinal details.The various implementation methods are:

- **Eucalyptus Cloud:** Eucalyptus is the open source Infrastructure as a service (IaaS) platform provides on demand access to the cloud. The eucalyptus consists of various components cloud controller, walrus for the data storage, Node controller, storage controller and cluster controller. The eucalyptus cloud is now acquired by the Hewlett Packard. Creating the eucalyptus environment is difficult. Once the test bed is created any cloud services can be implemented. The Access policy can be written and checked the correctness of the policy. The broker service is also available in eucalyptus cloud. The minimum requirement includes at least 4GB RAM and 2 Giga Hz processor. Thus the private cloud is created and using the cloud broker services the interoperability is achieved in the cloud. The software Defined Architecture (SDN) or the Network switch is to be used to connect the system. The IP addresses are checked dynamically by the broker services and transfer of the data takes place.
- **Open-Stack:** The open stack is again the private cloud supports IaaS. The open stack can be extended to the cloud federation using the emulator called Open-Day light. Compared to eucalyptus cloud the open stack is easy to deploy and test. The Open-Day light is used as emulator (brokerage) connecting the two private clouds. The usage of proxy servers is appreciated as the data are being outsourced outside the private cloud organization. Thus security and attacks needs to be monitored with secure Virtual Private Network (VPN). By means of using VPN increases the cost of the system.
- **Open Nebula and Comet Cloud:** The open nebula is a platform for creating the private cloud and supports the interoperability [5]. The comet cloud is the framework for the autonomic provisioning of the cloud federation. And it

supports the dynamic provisioning and secure data transfer and programming support for the inter-operability. The comet cloud framework will overcome the federation policy.

All the three open source Cloud Infrastructure support are well compatible with Amazon Cloud services.

CONCLUSION AND FUTURE DIRECTION

As every domain is being converted from the Traditional computing to the cloud computing and rapid increase in cloud services makes the CISCO to shift from networking domain to the private cloud. And initiated the Inter-cloud project in the year 2011. The CISCO has not invested such a huge money in any project so far. Nearly 2 billion USD has been spent. By deploying the cloud service with standards makes the secure data transfer. Thus we have proposed a hypothesis regarding cloud federation and architecture with suitable implementation module for health cloud. Our proposed work overcomes the various limitation of cloud. And also it paves the way for future cloud-health solutions by moving to multi-cloud scenario. With such an expectation among clients for a federated cloud it is only a matter of time its applications become more and more useful. One of the prominent use of federation is in big data analytics. With such huge network of interconnected and interoperable clouds from various providers' analysis of data in them will produce tremendous changes in today's business environment. With such a varied data better inference can be gathered and surveys can be conducted. And these cloud can communicate across multiple geographical locations. Thus an autonomous federated cloud is highly appealing. So a cloud federation can help client is making better use of technologies and provides confidence for client to turn towards cloud technologies.

REFERENCES

An Efficient Framework and Access Control Scheme for Cloud Health Care. (2015). In *Proceedings of IEEE 7th International Conference on Cloud Computing Technology and Science (CloudCom)*. Vancouver, Canada: IEEE.

Balamurugan, B., Krishna, P. V., Kumar, N. S., & Rajyalakshmi, G. V. (2015). An Efficient Framework for Health System Based on Hybrid Cloud with ABE-Outsourced Decryption. In *Artificial Intelligence and Evolutionary Algorithms in Engineering Systems* (pp. 41–49). Springer India. doi:10.1007/978-81-322-2135-7_6

Balamurugan, B., Krishna, P. V., Rajya Lakshmi, G. V., & Kumar, N. S. (2014, July). Cloud cluster communication for critical applications accessing C-MPICH. In *Embedded Systems (ICES), 2014 International Conference on* (pp. 145-150). IEEE.

Balamurugan, B., Kumar, N. S., Lakshmi, G. V., & Shanmuga, R. N. S. (2014, November). Common Cloud Architecture for Cloud Interoperability. In *Proceedings of the 2014 International Conference on Information and Communication Technology for Competitive Strategies* (p. 10). ACM.

Balamurugan, B., & Kumar, S. (2013). Enhancing privacy in cloud using Attribute Based Encryption. In *International Conference on Mathematical Computer Engineering-ICMCE* (p. 641).

Balamurugan, B., Venkata Krishna, P., Rajya, L. G., & Saravana Kumar, N. (2014, May). Layered storage architecture for health system using cloud. In *Advanced Communication Control and Computing Technologies (ICACCCT), 2014 International Conference on* (pp. 1795-1800). IEEE. doi:10.1109/ICACCCT.2014.7019419

Bethencourt, J., Sahai, A., & Waters, B. (2007). Ciphertext-policy attributebased encryption. In *Security and Privacy, SP '07. IEEE Symposium on*, (pp. 321–334). IEEE.

Dikaiakos, M. D., Katsaros, D., Mehra, P., Pallis, G., & Vakali, A. (2009). Cloud computing: Distributed internet computing for IT and scientific research. *IEEE Internet Computing*, *13*(5), 10–13. doi:10.1109/MIC.2009.103

Krutz, R. L., & Vines, R. D. (2010). *Cloud security: A comprehensive guide to secure cloud computing*. Wiley Publishing.

Kumar, N. S., Lakshmi, G. R., & Balamurugan, B. (2015). Enhanced Attribute Based Encryption for Cloud Computing. *Procedia Computer Science*, *46*, 689–696. doi:10.1016/j.procs.2015.02.127

Lai, Deng, Guan, & Weng. (2013). Attribute-based encryption with verifiable outsourced decryption. *IEEE Transactions on Information Forensics and Security*, *8*(8), 1343–1354.

Ortiz, S. Jr. (2011). The problem with cloud-computing standardization. *Computer*, *44*(7), 13–16. doi:10.1109/MC.2011.220

Poddar, R., Vishnoi, A., & Mann, V. (2015, January). HAVEN: Holistic load balancing and auto scaling in the cloud. In *Communication Systems and Networks (COMSNETS), 2015 7th International Conference on* (pp. 1-8). IEEE.

Toosi, A. N., Calheiros, R. N., & Buyya, R. (2014). *Interconnected cloud computing environments: Challenges, taxonomy, and survey. In ACM Computing Surveys*. CSUR.

Chapter 4
An Adaptive Cloud Proto Type Model for Health Care System:
An Adaptive Cloud Proto Type Model for Health Care System Using Software Defined Network (SDN)

Drashti Dave
Central University of Rajasthan, India

Nagaraju Aitha
Central University of Rajasthan, India

ABSTRACT

In the current Information Technology virtualization is one of the key components during the performance evaluation of network enabled environment including distributed computing, cloud computing, grid computing or pervasive computing. The network administrators and forensic teams are working on software defined networking (SDN) using which the network components can be controlled and managed using virtual infrastructure and global view of the physical network. On the physical implementation viewpoint, the single error or oversight can be damage the entire network integration. Now days, the advent of SDN products are being used in the research, development and corporate industry so that the effective control including routing, scheduling, security and related algorithms can be implemented

DOI: 10.4018/978-1-5225-1002-4.ch004

on real networks. There are number of real life applications where the software defined networking and service oriented architecture (SOA) can be implemented for the social and global cause. Medical and Health Care Service is one of the key domain can make use SDN approach in which the number of medical decisions are to be taken based availability of the enterprise information. In this research work, the case analysis and a prototype for health care management service is accomplished. In this chapter, a unique and pragmatic implementation of the SDN based on virtualization is done and the prototype which we proposed in this chapter will be validated in future by using mininet-openflow integration to evaluate the performance of network and data packets transmission.

that a controller communicates with network devices in SDN architecture. It was proposed to enable researchers to test new ideas in a production environment [6,7,8].

Open Flow provides the migration layer for control logic from a switch into the controller. It presents a protocol for the effective communication between controller and network switches [9,10].

Software Defined Networks (SDN) is an emerging technology nowadays to improve the speed of the data transmission. The main idea of this work is to integrate the hospitals under the same organization which is to share the information through SDN protocol architecture. The proposed model could work as a special case in medical field to share the experiences of doctors. The relevant information would be helpful to doctors as well as for patients. In the recent Information Technology well known social networking is highly crucial in day to day life. The proposed model could give expected results.

The underline LAN architecture may not perform well in integration switches and routers. Once the information is available in the remote sites the sharing of it is a crucial task. The sharing of the information will be performed well with SDN architecture. Security is a predominant factor in software defined networks (SDN), once the medical data is kept on the web then one can provide high level security to the applications developed with the medical data.

Figure 1 shows SDN architecture which shows the three-layer architecture which consisting of Infrastructure Layer, Control Layer and Application Layer. The open Flow protocol suite is an interface between Data plane (Infrastructure Layer) and Control Layer. The Control Layer generates the rules to forward the rules for data packets. A novel protocol suite is highly essential to maintain the security between Control and Infrastructure layer.

REVIEW OF EXISTING LITERATURE

To propose and defend the research work, a number of research papers are analyzed. Following are the excerpts from the different research work performed by number of academicians and researchers.

Adrian Laraet. al. (2014) : In this research manuscript, OpenFlow-based applications are proposed for the ease of network configuration for simplification of the network management. It is done by adding the security layers to virtualizethe networks as well as data centers and for deploying the mobile systems. Such applications can be executed on the top of operating systems including Beacon, Maestro, Floodlight, Nox, Trema or Node Flow. This study calculated the performance of Open Flow networks using modeling and experimentation. The work depicts the challenges which are faced by the large scale deployment of Open Flow-based networks.

Keisuke Nagase (2013) : Not just ordinary PC framework (i.e. Electric Medical Record, Physician Order section, PACS), additionally other restorative gear including ECG, US, EEG, X-beam and numerous others, are on-line now. Broad utilization of PC system intensifies unpredictability of programming PC system hardware. While medicinal services administration turns out to be more reliant on data innovation, such many-sided quality can bring about system disappointment that intrudes on wellbeing administration. As of late, idea of Software Defined Network (SDN) has

Figure 1. Software defined networking [2]

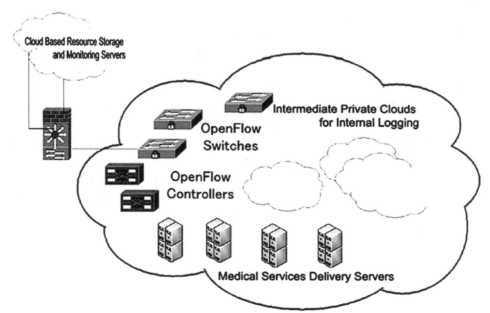

generally been acknowledged by system gear supplier and generation quality system hardware showed up in the business sector. SDN is an idea of programmable PC system fabric, as it was, system that can be powerfully reconfigured by downloading the settings from the controlling PC. This paper presented SDN in a healing facility system to assess its utility and security. After presentation of SDN, SDN section ended up being steady, and programmed rerouting maintaining a strategic distance from fizzled course was far speedier than routine innovation. The conclusion in this exploration paper is SDN is exceptionally significant innovation in medicinal services that is 24hr/365day mission basic business.

Shie-Yuan Wanget. al. (2013) : In this work, the authors introduces the EstiNet OpenFlow network simulator and emulator. The work presents he support for testing the functions and evaluating the performances of software-defined networks' Open-Flow controller's application programs. The simulator makes use of a kernel that is unique reentering simulation methodology to enable unmodified real applications to run on nodes inits simulated network. In thiswork, authors compare the EstiNet with ns-3 and Mininet regarding their capabilities, performance, and scalability.

Shimonishiet. al. (2012) : This paper clarifies the execution parts of OpenFlow and how it is utilized for system inquires about and tests, and in addition programming stage for that. OpenFlow has been proposed as a method for specialists, system administration inventors, and others to effortlessly plan, test, and convey their imaginative thoughts in trial or creation systems to quicken research exercises on wired or remote system advancements. As opposed to having programmability inside of every system hub, the isolated OpenFlow controller gives system control through pluggable programming modules. In this paper, the work presents the OpenFlow programming system Trema, which concentrates on efficiency of system investigations and spreads a whole improvement cycle of programming, testing, troubleshooting, and organization. This exploration paper presents some of our analyses including consistent handover in the middle of WiFi and WiMAX, multicast feature spilling, and system access control.

Bob Lantz et. al. (2010) : In this work, the authors share the supporting case studies culled from over100 users, at 18 institutions, who have developed Software-Defined Networks (SDN). Finally, the work reflects the greatest value of Mininet will be supporting collaborative network research, by enabling self-contained SDN prototypes which anyone with a PC can download, run, evaluate, explore, tweak, and build upon.

PROBLEM FORMULATION AND RESEARCH OBJECTIVES

The existing implementations of the classical virtualization and network components management in a grid and distributed environment are very complex and less cost effective. In this chapter as a case study the proposed model would be applied in health care situation. The proposed model can be applicable for a group of medical servers integrated with SDN architecture. The proposed model will be helpful to share the information among the group of hospitals. The architecture proposed in this chapter will work as prototype model for future SDN. As the cost is directly associated with the turnaround time and complexity, it is very important to keep track of these issues to overcome the flaws in network infrastructure management.

There is the need of software defined networking using which the complete set of network components can be managed with efficiency and overall cost factor can be reduced a lot.

Following are the research objectives in this work which are accomplished the simulation.

• To evaluate the performance of SDN suite and associated virtualization
• To perform the experiments on varying number of nodes and network devices
• To calculate and analyze the turnaround time and round trap time in each simulation iteration so that the effectiveness can be measured.

The concept is quite new and this chapter suggesting enabling SDN architecture to hospitals under the same organization or those hospitals would like to share the information. The SDN architecture would provide fast information processing from one node to another node. The open flow is protocol architecture which would enable virtualization within the existing network. The virtualization will be more beneficial while generating the rules. The generated rules enable the data transmission from one node to another node. The proposed chapter would suggest all the existing hospitals would be converting it into SDN technology while transmitting the data.

The Proposed Model

Security is the major concern and aspect that is mandatory for any network infrastructure. In SDN, as each and everything is dependent on the software and APIs part, it becomes necessary to enhance the layers of APIs and libraries so that any third party application or sniffer is not able to penetrate into the network.

In the SDN based architecture, following points should be considered and empowered so that the higher layers of security and privacy can be implemented

1. Security of the Controller against sniffing attacks to escalate the quality of service
2. Protecting the SDN Controller against DDoS Attacks for higher availability of the network
3. Establishment of the Trust Architecture so that authenticated and genuine nodes can transmit the data as well as signals
4. Creation of Robust and Strong Policy Guidelines as well Frameworks
5. Incorporation of the Forensics as well as Remediation Measures to detect and push back any attack

The Figure 2 is the proposed model which is secure mode SDN Frame work, in the proposed work Data Plane and Control Plane is separated. The Proposed work executes or run control plane software on hardware which can ensure the proper utilization of the existing hardware. The SDN decouple from the specific networking hardware from the existing network. The proposed work uses the existing servers and switches in more effective way. The data plane is programmable data plane which can allow flexible data forwarding plane. Maintain, control and program data plane state from a central entity is possible. Architecture to control not just a networking device but an entire network. The proposed model would try to propose models which overcome the packet delays so the fast packet forwarding is possible from source to destination. In the literature two-layer open flow protocols are advisable for packet forwarding. The first layer classifies the packet and the second layer forward the packet from source node to destination. The classification could be done in various ways one can do research to adopt different types of classifiers.

In the above figure controller will generate the rules to forward the packets. Here we can follow the different type of security policies. The police would be same for each flow. The syntax of the flow provides security policy to the packets. In the proposed work two kinds of APIs are available Northbound API and Southbound API. The control to Application Layer API we call it as Northbound API and Controller to switch we call it as Southbound API. The south bound API decides the flow controls which try to balance the load among the filter switches. The proposed models try to work different kinds of load balancing and novel packet forwarding algorithm from one node to another node with the help of dummy switches.

PROPOSED WORK AND IMPLEMENTATION

The proposed work will be implementing windows 7 (Host Operating System) and Ubuntu 14.04 (Guest OS) to implement the above proposed model. Mininet, Open Flow and POX Controller has been decided to use the proposed work. The Figure

Figure 2. Proposed SDN environment in secured mode

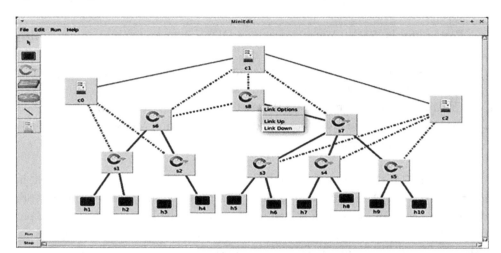

3 shows the Graphical User Interface (GUI) of Minnet Simulator which shows the SDN Frame work with virtual switches. The python scripts are useful to enable the rules to incorporate between the controller and filter switches.

The above Figure 4 Shows the scenario of the components which shows medical service open flow controllers and open flow enabled switches to forward the packets from source node to destination node. The above Figure 4 shows the cloud enable servers which can attract the huge traffic from the internet. Those servers could run different type of applications. The similar kinds of application generate the similar traffic flow. The open flow specifications have to generate the rules for the traffic which are of same class same rule has to generate.

Following tools are used for implementation of the complete virtualization scenario

1. Windows 7 (Host OS)
2. putty (SSH Client)
3. Ubuntu 14.04 (Guest OS)
4. Oracle VirtualBox (Installation of Guest OS)
5. MiniNet 2.2.1
6. OpenFlow based protocols which are controllers.

The above tools are essential tools to install Mininet emulator. The Emulator can be used to test the performance of open flow based protocols.

Figure 3. Connectivity of node with OpenFlow switch with controller

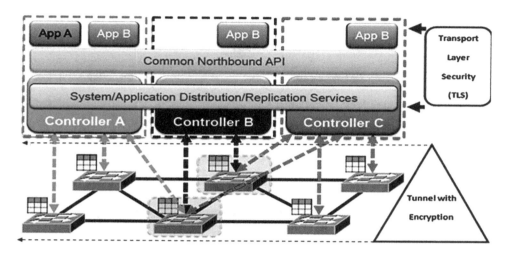

CASE ANALYSIS AND IMPLEMENTATION: HEALTH AND MEDICAL CARE

In our Virtualization enabled hospital automation, the case of anesthesia injection in the hospital operation theatres is taken. Suppose there are 10 operation theaters in a hospital and each block needs the anesthesia injection to some extent by taking the constraint of limited anesthesia in the hospital. These 10 hospitals have been connected with switches and controllers, So the hospitals share the information through the controllers and switches. The proposed model could develop two layer protocols which improve the connectivity among the hospitals through virtual topology.

If a particular operation theatre needs more delivery, the server (controller) will analyze the requirements depending upon assorted parameters of the patient including blood pressure and other aspects. The server (controller) will decide whether to deliver that anesthesia or to provide the alternate resource.

Pseudo Code

1. Activate and Initialized the Server (Controller) C_i
2. Activate and Initialized the Intermediate Load Balancers (Switches) S_i
3. Generate the Delivery Points (Operation Theatres) h_i
4. in each h_i
   a. h_1 initiates the request R_j to specific injection to be injected from the server point

Figure 4. Set up scenario of the components

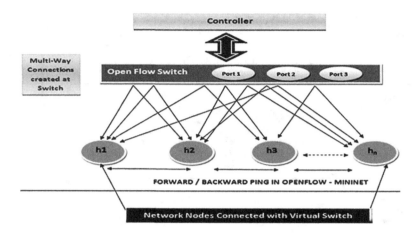

    b.   for each R_j, Si will forward the request to C_i

    c.   if $R>A_j$ (A_j -> Available Injection) deliver alternate resource else $R_j :=$ h_1 (Delivery to be implemented)

5.   Analyze the Log Reports of each $h_i S_i$ matrix

The proposed case scenario and implementation is done on Hospital ICU Automation in which there are number of delivery points of the services and a centralized server from where the resources will be transmitted.

Components of the Proposed Hospital System with Virtualization

1.   Centralized Server with Sub-Controllers (c0-c2)
2.   Intermediate Modules for Load Balancing and Routing (s1 - s8)
3.   Operation Theatres (h1-h10)

CONCLUSION

With the use of software defined networking (SDN), the actual implementation and management of the network infrastructure is made easy. The base technologies behind the scenario are the virtualization and remote clients. The proposed method would be helpful to share the information among the group of hospitals. The proposed model will be implemented using Mininet Emulator. The case study will be executed in the proposed environment. The proposed model would be executed with the defined scenario. The proposed model would enhance the packet delivery and packet throughput among the hosts. Recently authors are proposing two layer open flow based switches. The proposed work enhances the performance of the existing protocols.

REFERENCES

Azodolmolky, S. (2013). *Software Defined Networking with OpenFlow*. Packt Publishing Ltd.

Boughzala, B., Ben Ali, R., Lemay, M., Lemieux, Y., & Cherkaoui, O. (2011, May). OpenFlow supporting inter-domain virtual machine migration. In *Wireless and Optical Communications Networks (WOCN), 2011 Eighth International Conference on* (pp. 1-7). IEEE. doi:10.1109/WOCN.2011.5872945

Kim, H., Kim, J., & Ko, Y. B. (2014, February). Developing a cost-effective OpenFlow-testbed for small-scale Software Defined Networking. In *Advanced Communication Technology (ICACT), 2014 16th International Conference on* (pp. 758-761). IEEE.

Lantz, B., Heller, B., & McKeown, N. (2010, October). A network in a laptop: rapid prototyping for software-defined networks. In *Proceedings of the 9th ACM SIGCOMM Workshop on Hot Topics in Networks* (p. 19). ACM. doi:10.1145/1868447.1868466

Lara, A., Kolasani, A., & Ramamurthy, B. (2014). Network innovation using open-flow: A survey. *IEEE Communications Surveys and Tutorials*, *16*(1), 493–512. doi:10.1109/SURV.2013.081313.00105

McKeown, N., Anderson, T., Balakrishnan, H., Parulkar, G., Peterson, L., Rexford, J., & Turner, J. et al. (2008). Openflow: Enabling innovation in campus networks. *SIGCOMM Comput. Commun. Rev.*, *38*(2), 69–74. doi:10.1145/1355734.1355746

Msahli, M., Pujolle, G., Serrhrouchni, A., Fadlallah, A., & Guenane, F. (2012, November). Openflow and on demand Networks. In *Network of the Future (NOF), 2012 Third International Conference on the* (pp. 1-5). IEEE. doi:10.1109/NOF.2012.6464006

Salsano, S., Ventre, P. L., Prete, L., Siracusano, G., Gerola, M., & Salvadori, E. (2014, September). OSHI-Open Source Hybrid IP/SDN networking (and its emulation on Mininet and on distributed SDN testbeds). In *Software Defined Networks (EWSDN), 2014 Third European Workshop on* (pp. 13-18). IEEE.

Tourrilhes, J., Sharma, P., Banerjee, S., & Pettit, J. (2014). SDN and OpenFlow Evolution: A Standards Perspective. *Computer*, *47*(11), 22–29. doi:10.1109/MC.2014.326

Wang, S. Y. (2014, June). Comparison of SDN OpenFlow network simulator and emulators: EstiNet vs. Mininet. In *Computers and Communication (ISCC), 2014 IEEE Symposium on* (pp. 1-6). IEEE.

Chapter 5
Big Data Analytics for Childhood Pneumonia Monitoring

Suresh Kumar Peddoju
Kakatiya Institute of Technology and Science, India

Kavitha K.
Indian Institute of Technology, India

Sharma S. C.
Indian Institute of Technology, India

ABSTRACT

In developing countries pediatric pneumonia is the second leading cause of deaths and 98% of pneumonia-induced deaths are identified across the world. It is mandatory to identify the symptoms of pneumonia in children to avoid mortality causing complications. Early identification of children at risk for treatment failure or at increased risk for death will help to improve overall health outcomes. If pneumonia is suspected, it is important to seek medical attention promptly so that an accurate diagnosis can be made and appropriate treatment is given in time. The proposed approach quickly provides history of previous patient's details, expert doctor's opinions who are in globe and their previous treatment for the same symptoms, all diagnostic reports such as blood tests, x-ray etc., from the cloud and gives analytics from big data to take fast and precise decisions by the doctors.

DOI: 10.4018/978-1-5225-1002-4.ch005

INTRODUCTION

The developing countries face many risks and obstacles for giving timely and appropriate treatment for children with pneumonia leading globally to child deaths of 1 million approximately. Childhood pneumonia is the second leading cause of deaths amongst children globally; in specific 98% of pneumonia-induced deaths (UNICEF Report) occur in developing countries. It is important to recognize how pneumonia symptoms show up in children in order to avoid any life-threatening complications. Children were at greater risk of contracting the disease because their immune system is not fully developed. Early identification of children at risk for treatment failure or at increased risk for deaths will help improve overall health outcomes. If pneumonia is suspected, it is important to seek medical attention promptly so that an accurate diagnosis can be made and appropriate treatment can be given in time. The doctor will take a medical history and will conduct a diagnostic test to find severity of the condition of patient to give appropriate antibiotics/medicines timely for effective and immediate treatment.

The motive of this chapter is learning the things from the past will give better results for future. Now-a-days healthcare data is very large, critical and more complex. According to World Wide Web, healthcare data across the world is expected to reach 25,000 petabytes in 2020. The average healthcare spending of all the countries especially India per year accounts about 25% in the country overall GDP. Even after spending much amount for healthcare, the average life expectancy of all the countries (including developed and developing) is all about 70-75 years (Eg., India-65 yrs, UK-80 yrs, Germany-82 yrs, Japan-83 yrs, Poland-76 yrs etc.,) only.

Over 30 billion dollars were spent on hospital admissions which are unnecessary. We can reduce these unnecessary hospital admissions by identifying patients who are at high-risk and ensure they should get the appropriate treatment in time. New strategies should be evolved to identify the patient's health status well before it's too late for treatment and needs hospital admission. By this way we can reduce number of unnecessary hospital admissions. If we could able to identify the health condition of the patient primarily, then new algorithms will predict the status of patient health and need of hospital admission can be suggested to the doctor. Based on these inputs doctor suggests need of hospital admission and by this way there is decrease in healthcare cost. Regular re-admission into hospitals is harmful and cost effective. In case of heart attack, heart failure etc., especially childhood pneumonia patients get admitted into hospitals in regular intervals due to poor care after previous discharge.

This proposal is coining to save the child from Pneumonia by designing and developing an effective, efficient and timely treatment mechanism using latest technologies such as Mobile Cloud and Big Data Analytics.

Objectives

The objectives of proposed approach presented in this chapter are as follows:

- The motive of this proposed approach is to recognize the pneumonia symptoms in a child well before and identifying patients at risk of admission into hospitals.
- This approach will help the doctors in taking appropriate decisions for giving better treatment at right time.
- Digitization of patient's data should be done to store it in cloud for anywhere, anytime availability and can be accessed by any one.
- Estimating the severity level of the pneumonia disease by analyzing and accessing different patients data from cloud and provide best possible suggestions for the doctors to treat the child effectively, efficiently and timely.
- Different kinds of data (may be structured and unstructured) such as diagnosis reports, blood test reports and x-ray of pneumonia patients which can becomes big data, should be analyzed by using big data analytics techniques.
- Trustworthiness of doctor's information can be evaluated and if any false updations were done by fraudulent doctors can be identified to block/eliminate such doctor's suggestions.
- This proposed approach guide how efficiently uses resources and can potentially save millions of healthcare dollars each year.
- Effectively integrating and efficiently analyzing various forms of healthcare data over a period of time can answer many of the impending healthcare problems.

BACKGROUND

According to The United Nations Children's Fund (UNICEF) estimation pneumonia is about to kill 3 million children every year. Although most fatalities occur in developing countries, pneumonia remains a significant cause of morbidity in industrialized nations. The most frequent cause of morbidity among children is lower respiratory tract infection. Of these infections pneumonia predicts as the most serious disease and can be hard to diagnose (Mccracken et al., 2000). According to World Health Organization (WHO), 2-3 million deaths occur per year occur in children less than 5 years old due to pneumonia. From the history of over last decade, a vast quantity of studies shows lack in the diagnosis and management of childhood pneumonia in the developing countries where the young children and infants leading to death.

Childhood Pneumonia

Pneumonia is usually caused due to infection of viruses, fungi, bacteria or parasites. It is primarily characterized by the inflammation of the lung tissue especially alveoli filled with water. Alveoli are the microscopic sacs in the lungs that absorb oxygen. Pneumonia is different and more severe when compared to bronchitis which is characterized by the inflammation of the large airways, the bronchi caused due to the infection. In some cases, pneumonia and bronchitis may appear together named as bronchopneumonia. Most of the pneumonia cases studied was the infections caused by the bacterial group called atypical. Pneumonia occurs when a germ (bacteria or virus or fungi or protozoan) through breathing enter into the body of poor health or low immunity. Pneumonia is a common cause of death in people especially children who are already unwell. Pneumonia claims the life of a child every 20 seconds. While 98 percent of pneumonia-induced deaths occur in developing countries, it's still important to recognize how its symptoms show up in children in order to avoid any life-threatening complications. Most of the people due to ill health require hospital admission.

Symptoms

Cough and cold, high temperature, shivering, not willing to take food, headaches and other body pains, making more sputum colored green or yellow or sometimes bloodstained, unable to breathe, fast breath developing a tight chest, if pleura (a layer between the lung and the chest wall) also get infected, a sharp pain in the side of the chest may develop which can be identified by listening a crackle sound using stethoscope by a doctor. Pneumonia symptoms may differ according to the age. Adults affected with pneumonia show the following symptoms like feeling of short breath, pain during cough and pain in the chest. In the case of infants and children symptoms are less specific and clear signs of chest infection may not appear. Instead they also show high temperature, appearing unwell and appear lethargic. Skin, lips and nail beds may sometimes become dark or bluish which indicates lungs disfunctioning in the supply of adequate oxygen to the body. At this stage immediate medical assistance is required.

Diagnosis

If pneumonia is suspected, it is important to seek medical attention promptly so that an accurate diagnosis can be made and appropriate treatment given. The doctor will take a medical history and will conduct a physical examination. During the examination the doctor will listen to the chest with a stethoscope. Coarse breathing, crackling sounds, wheezing and reduced breath sounds in a particular part of the lungs can indicate pneumonia. In order to confirm the diagnosis a chest x-ray is usually taken. The x-ray will show the area of the lung affected by the pneumonia. Blood tests may also be taken and a sample of the sputum may be sent to the laboratory for testing.

Differential Diagnosis

The primary step in diagnosing pediatric pneumonia is physical examination of the child's respiratory effort. Table 1 shows the threshold values for identifying children with pneumonia given by the World Health Organization (WHO) are as follows:

If any respiratory symptoms are observed, then assessment of oxygen saturation is performed by pulse oximetry. Sometimes in severe cases in order to detect cyanosis cyanography is conducted to evaluate children with potential respiratory compromise. Culturing of samples, serum testing, complete blood picture count, chest scanning and ultrasonography are the other diagnostic tests may be included.

Depending upon the range of symptoms shown by the patient, pneumonia vary from mild to severe and even life threatening.

Mild Pneumonia in Children

Certain bacteria like Mycoplasma pneumoniae and Chlamydophila pneumoniae cause mild symptoms which leads to mild pneumonia. This pneumonia is also known as walking or atypical pneumonia as it is more common in school-age children. Symptoms shown by this pneumonia are dry cough, tiredness, low grade fever and headache.

Moderate Pneumonia in Children

Pneumonia caused by viruses show moderate pneumonia mostly in preschool children between 4 months and 5 years old. Children affected by this pneumonia, show symptoms such as cough, low grade fever, sore throat, loss of appetite, nasal congestion, diarrhea, lack of energy and feeling tiredness.

Severe Pneumonia in Children

The most common type of pneumonia affected by the school age children and teens is caused by bacteria is called severe pneumonia. Symptoms of this type of

Table 1. Threshold values for identifying children with pneumonia

Children at Age in Months	Number of Breaths/ Minute
<2	≥ 60
2 – 11	≥ 50
12 – 59	≥ 40

pneumonia show abrupt conditions such as high fever, wheezing, cough producing green or yellowish mucus, flushed skin, difficulty in breathing, chills or sweating, a bluish tint to the lips or nail beds. Children affected with pneumonia feel sicker.

Other Symptoms of Pneumonia

It is difficult to identify the new born or infants affected with pneumonia as they do not show any typical signs of pneumonia infection. Determination becomes tricky as they may not be able to communicate how they suffer as an older child can. The symptoms indicate that an infant or a young child is suffering from pneumonia are feeding poorly, crying more than usual, looking pale, vomiting, feeling lethargic and being restless or irritable.

Healthcare Data

Health care data refers to electronic health record of a patient. It is large and complex that it is very hard to manage with existing and common data management methods (Priyanka & Kulennavar, 2014). The data generated by different devices such as wearables or sensors may be collected and analyzed in real-time.

Categories of data in healthcare:

1. **Genomic Data:** Genomic data is about genetic organisms of patients. This data will contain DNA and RNA codes, sequencing of codes, mapping of codes and analyzing the codes (Chen et al., 2012). Genomics generates vast volumes of data; each patient genome has approximately 25,000 genes.
2. **Clinical Data:** Clinical data is enormously used in healthcare and medical research. This data can be gathered at the time of patient care or as part of sampling or trail purpose. Clinical data which includes laboratory data such as blood samples, serum samples, urine samples etc., and electronic medical records (EMR) come under structured data (Yang et al., 2014). The data which includes post-op notes, patient discharge card which gives summary of ongoing treatment undergone during admission, X-ray and all other scanning reports and images come under unstructured data.
3. **Patient Behavior Data:** Now-a-days people are searching for a solution in an easy and faster way by browsing the web. During this process, patients can find relevant information regarding their disease by browsing search engines, taking opinions from people by using social networks such as twitter, Facebook, whatsup, healthplan professionals etc., (Terry, 2013).
4. **Healthcare Publication and Clinical Reference Data:** The research publications such as journals, medical reference materials come under healthcare

     publication data and publications related to clinical references about drug information under clinical reference data (Miller, 2012).

5. **Administrative, Business and External Data:** Administrative related information such as financial reports, billing information, scheduling (Terry, 2013) and all insurance claims data should also be maintained. The employees such as doctor's, staff and other staff finger prints, iris information and related information is to be stored.

6. **Other Data:** The data related to patient's personal health records such as e-mails and the data communicated between the patient and provider should be stored. Device generated data, adverse events and feedback (Yang et al., 2014) given by different patients or consumers of the healthcare applications should be maintained.

CLOUD COMPUTING IN HEALTHCARE

Cloud computing is an interconnected network of different kinds of devices which will deliver different services such as software-as-a-service, platform-as-a-service and Infrastructure-as-a-service. The basic characteristics of cloud are on-demand, elastic, pay-as-you-use and resource sharing. The users connected to cloud can acquire the services on-demand and they can increase or decrease the resources as per their financial concerns. Virtualization is the basic principle behind cloud for providing different cloud offerings timely and efficiently. Globally distributed healthcare organizations are adopting cloud-based services for storing their patient's information in cloud. In coming days, cloud usage will increase to run their healthcare applications by healthcare organizations.

Every hospital across the countries is digitizing patient's data, which requires on-demand infrastructure services. Healthcare organizations are accelerating migration of their information to cloud. Healthcare is moving to a digital platform and it becoming more patient-centric and data-driven. Large international players such as Microsoft, Qualcomm Life, Philips, Verizon and AT&T have launched cloud-based vertical solutions aimed at the healthcare sector, and the global trend is that cloud solutions are supporting greater sharing and accessibility of health data. Cloud computing can share healthcare data between different parties through secured mechanisms such as encryption and tokenization of data at rest, in transit and in process.

Despite the fact that the concept of cloud computing is not new, it is only recently that cloud technologies and applications are widespread (Jennings, 2009; Vaquero et al., 2008; Velte et al., 2010). Cloud computing offers the potential to dramatically reduce the cost of software services through the commoditization of IT assets and on-demand usage patterns. According to the Gartner senior analyst Ben Pring (2011) "it's become the phrase du jour". Virtualization of hardware, rapid service provisioning, scalability, elasticity, accounting, granularity and cost allocation models allow clouds to promise the ability to efficiently integrate and adapt resource provisioning to the dynamic demands of end users and applications (Chorafas, 2011; Dillon et al., 2010; Doukas et al., 2010; Marks, 2008; Rittinghouse and Ransome, 2009). Following this stream of motivation, more and more vendors are offering healthcare solutions and services such as telemedicine, electronic medical records, medical imaging, and patient management that can be consumed or integrated by healthcare providers, payers and customers over a cloud.

State of the art technologies like cloud computing and SOA are used to provide efficient, scalable, portable, interoperable and integrated IT infrastructures that are cost effective and maintainable. As explained despite the significant importance of these technologies, the healthcare sector is just starting to realize their potential. As a result, many standalone applications exist in the area of healthcare which providing services and supporting the activities of all actors involved, such as, patients, healthcare professionals, laboratories, hospitals etc. Due to the non-integrated nature of e-healthcare applications and services numerous medical errors occur that cause the death of thousands of patients per year. For that reason, it is of high importance to integrate healthcare services into cloud. In addition to this, there is a need to deliver better services and reduce the cost of health expenses. The latter can be achieved through patient monitoring of applications that will allow patients to continue their treatment at home and will free up space and staff at hospitals. All these can be realized through an innovative integrated e-health services platform that utilizes advanced technologies like cloud computing and SOA.

BIG DATA IN HEALTHCARE

Now-a-days every hospital is maintaining the patient medical health record and terabytes of patient data is to be stored in server. In that 80% of data is image data like CT scan, ECG, MRI and X-rays which are of unstructured data. The medical image data is Big Data which is huge in size, highly complex and multi-dimensional. Big Data can be used to predict health risks of patient and improve clinical treatment. Approximately four hundred and fifty billion dollars can be saved in healthcare domain by using Big Data.

Big Data Challenges in Healthcare Domain

1. Inferring knowledge from diverse set of healthcare repositories which consists of patient history, diagnostic reports, prescribed medication, vital signs and progress notes of patients (White, 2014).
2. Aggregation, consolidation and analysis of unstructured data such as scanned documents, images, diagnostic reports etc., is very difficult. Effective extraction of relevant information can be achieved from large volumes of unstructured data within a right context is a foremost challenge.
3. Genomic data is critical in its nature for analyzing and it also much difficult to combine genomics with clinical data. This task is computationally complex and it is a very critical challenge.
4. Telemetry data generated from different automated monitoring sensors is another challenge in healthcare domain. The data collected from several sensors for blood pressure, glucose, weight and pulse oximetry etc., is complex (Halamka, 2014). Capturing of streaming temporal data is also another important challenge (Schultz, 2013).
5. Doctors are sparing their maximum time in finding the cause of the disease for better treatment. Big data is giving solution for it, but the data in medical repositories are huge in size, noisy in nature or may be false information (Bottles and Begoli, 2014). Identifying false information and getting trustworthy results is a next challenge.
6. Privacy issues related to patients data including health insurance is a barrier to big data (Warner, 2013). It is so difficult to maintain proper balance between patient's data and usage of algorithms on the data.
7. Protecting patient's data from data hacking and data leakages become more dangerous challenge with big data.
8. Shortfall of resources/infrastructure, policies and practices are the concerns for adopting big data.

Benefits of Big Data in Healthcare

1. Exact and precise diagnosis can be done, detection of patients who are at severe health risks can be identified and every patient health data can be customized accordingly. This can improve the overall outcome of health.
2. Early identification of diseases, removal of unnecessary and redundant admissions, changes in care will minimize the costs.
3. Foresee and managing different pathological conditions which are at risk.
4. Identifying the health care fraud more rapidly and efficiently based on huge amounts of historical data.

5.   By applying statistical models on medical data of individual patient can reduce unnecessary usage of emergency services and also provide the appropriate emergency services with lower cost in a minimum time.

6.   Different tools can be used to analyze the health data collected at multiple levels, such as molecular, tissue and patient information. The amount of data which is big in size can be produced by Health Informatics has grown day by day. Big Data analytics can be used to gain knowledge about health conditions of patient and can be treated timely and effectively.

Big Data Analytics

The usage of big data analytics in healthcare domain is in its immature stage needs to be further extended by applying innovative techniques. Healthcare domain generates huge amounts of data to become big data which needs applicability of big data analytics. The complexities in the big data can be sorted out by using analytics which will provide many more insights about the patient diagnosis or treatment related information in a right time with precise decisions. Big data analytics can be enormously applied on healthcare data to yield instant healthcare outcomes to decrease the healthcare costs.

Applications of Big Data in Healthcare Domain

- **Genomics Analytics:** Big data analytics can be applied on genomic data to provide much more efficient and precise treatment before the adverse health conditions arise like cancer etc., Genomic data alone is insufficient to maintain complete patient record, so by combining clinical data with patient's genomic data can resolve this problem and provide timely treatment to save the patient.

- **Flu Outbreak Prediction and Control:** Digitization of public health information become helpful to detect and manage potential disease out breaks by analyzing the public health data continuously. The information floating in web and social media should be analyzed by applying big data analytics to predict flu out breaks.

- **Clinical Outcome Analytics:** Different kinds of data like clinical, financial and operation should be analyzed for clinical decisions. Any disease can be identified and given better treatment based on the clinical decisions. Blue cross and Blue Shield of North Carolina, USA has applied different big data analytics to reduce the cost of healthcare and it also predicts health risks with improved clinical outcomes (Helm-Murtagh, 2014).

- **Fraud Detection and Prevention:** Big data analytics can be used to find fraud claims done by patients. If we apply analytics to claims data, then fraud claims can be identified and minimized to healthcare payers. Fraud waste and abuse analytics can be performed on this data to help the payers from financial loss (White, 2014).
- **Medical Device Design and Manufacturing:** Computational methods as well as big data analytics can be widely used in medical device design and manufacturing field (Erdman and Keefe, 2013) to set configurations, maintain device materials and other things.
- **Personalized Patient Care:** There are two popular models in healthcare domain; they are disease-centered and patient-centered model. Personalized patient care (Chawla N.V et al, 2013) can be done by creating personalized disease risk profile and disease management. This is the core area where big data analytics can be applied to assist and guide the personalized treatment to improve the overall health condition of the patient.
- **E-Consultation and Tele-Diagnosis:** E-consultation is upcoming area in healthcare domain where aggregated images and stream of data from different hospitals across worldwide is becoming big data and helping on-site practitioners to give appropriate treatment at right time. All the consultation data is integrated to store it in a cloud and by applying big data analytics we can predict 50% of the deaths due to high risk diseases. Authors of this chapter concentrated on this domain and proposed a novel approach for e-consultation and diagnosis the diseases with less time to save the child from pneumonia deaths.
- **Pharmaceuticals and Medicine:** Pharmaceutical industry data is becoming increasing day by day to become big data. This industry also needs big data analytics to manage pharmaceutical information as well as updation of medicine information. Drug discovery can be done by analyzing the data available in pharmaceutical industry to improve and manage medicine information to provide appropriate medicine to the patients without delays.
- **Smart Health and Wellbeing:** Big data analytics has huge opportunities in medical applications in specific smart health care. In present day of digitized world, hospitals are also digitized and telemedicine is so popular in wellbeing of patients.

TREATMENT FOR CHILDHOOD PNEUMONIA

Treating pneumonia depends on what caused the infection, and can range from outpatient treatment to surgery. But because the illness comes in different forms, treatment plans vary widely. Some may only need bed rest, while others may require hospitalization. Doctor will outline a plan that is specific to the condition of pneumonia, severe condition of patient, age, and overall health condition. And they also suggest patients that the place of treatment would be at home or hospital. He will also suggest whether patient needs antibiotics or not. Many children under the age of 12 will engage in something called "play therapy" with their therapist. Play therapy (in its varying forms) is a dynamic, creative, evidence based approach towards working with children.

Treatment at Home

If a person is normally well and pneumonia is not severe he can be treated at home based on the infected organism's etiology and the age and the clinical condition of the patient. Usually an antibiotic will be necessary for the complete cure of the pneumonia. For most of the pneumonia caused due to bacteria, antibiotic Amoxicillin is used as an effective drug and recovers the body within three days or if it persists longer than three weeks should consult a doctor again. Drinking lots of fluids to avoid dehydration and taking paracetomol at regular intervals to get rid from high temperature and body aches. These precautions must be taken while undergoing treatment at home. For children suspected with pneumonia should be primarily checked with pulse oximetry through which observe the respiratory complications and if needed oxygen should be supplied. Many children more than five years old do not require hospital admission as they respond well to the oral antibiotics.

Treatment at Hospital

If the pneumonia is severe or it's not cured within three weeks using oral antibiotics and also the person with poor health requires hospital admission. More often children less than 5 years of age require hospitalization depending upon their clinical status. A chest X-ray will confirm the presence of pneumonia, it also identifies the presence of effusion and range of infection. A short delay during administration or treating the patient may require longer durations of ventilation, complete hospitalization with ICU stay. Blood tests and sputum tests of the effected person will predict the type of infected bacteria and also helps to take specific antibiotic against it. Sometimes the supply of oxygen, intensive care unit and other supportive techniques are used depending on the person's health conditions. After the discharge from the hospital or by returning home the person may feel tired or sick for some time even though the treatment is completed.

CLOUD-BASED TREATMENT FOR CHILDHOOD PNEUMONIA

Cloud can be used to store any kind of data and can access any information from anywhere at any time. For this reason, the proposed approach is adopted cloud for the treatment of childhood pneumonia patients. The cloud can be used to interconnect all the doctors' information and used to store their diagnosis reports and treatment related information. This approach assumes that all the doctors, patients, staff as stakeholders of the cloud and who will disseminate information through the cloud. The motive for considering cloud-based treatment for childhood pneumonia is its rapid service provisioning and on-demand usage patterns.

The in-patient's and out-patient's information gathered in each hospital is stored in cloud and interconnectivity of all the hospitals data is integrated through cloud. The data stored in cloud can be shared to all the stakeholders of the cloud across the globe. Further, the health data of all the diseases in particularly pneumonia patient's data is stored in cloud and can be used by any doctor across the globe at any time. Due to this reason the proposed approach adopted cloud as a basis to store the childhood pneumonia patient's data. By doing in such a way any doctor can have access to this data for the best way to treat pneumonia. So that any doctor can give better treatment by choosing best possible solution from readily available solutions which are available at cloud. Through this best solution, doctors can take fast and precise decisions for treating the child who is having pneumonia in-time to save childhood deaths. Doctors can also share their opinions and views by updating information in the cloud regarding the health conditions, abnormal behavior of child with pneumonia and any other relevant information which they feel mandatory for further use.

Cloud is having vast information in it and the healthcare data is increasing day by day through different sources which are becoming Big Data. Due to digitization of doctor's and patient's data which include X-ray, blood test reports and other pathology reports are of different kinds like structured and unstructured. Accessing such unstructured vast variety of data and analyzing such big data requires efficient algorithms to acquire relevant data within short span of time. Due to this reason big data analytics are used in this proposed approach to dig the patient's data for acquiring relevant information to take right decisions at right time.

Security and Trust plays a significant role in distributed environment like cloud where highly dynamic sharing of resources is involved. There is always a threat of fraudulent parties to update information in cloud to create an unpredicted environment that may lead to adversity. In such unpredicted environment identifying the trustworthy doctor's data is a difficult task. The data updated by different doctors in cloud may or may not be trustworthy due to fraud doctor's information or false entry by the doctors. Identifying such untrustworthy doctor's data is a big challenge and giving right information by evaluating trustworthiness of doctor's data by calculating direct and indirect trust rating about those doctors. Further, estimating direct trust based on satisfaction of the doctors who are giving treatment to pneumonia patient. Indirect trust evaluation is influenced by various factors like the level of unreliable feedbacks and credibility of the recommenders (doctors and patients) recommendations. Based on the evaluation of trustworthiness of doctor's data, the fraudulent doctor's information is eliminated or blocked.

The proposed approach in this chapter quickly provides history of previous patient's details, expert doctors who are in globe and their previous treatment for the same symptoms, all diagnostic reports such as blood tests, x-ray etc., from the cloud and gives analytics from big data to take fast and precise decisions by the doctors.

The challenges encountered in this process are:

- Storing the patients records in a place like Cloud where they can be accessed from anywhere and anytime
- Accessing and analyzing different patient's data across the world to estimate the severity level of the disease and provide best possible solutions on the fly to treat the patients effectively and efficiently.
- Providing the easy to understand reporting mechanisms for browsing the results and understanding them thoroughly and immediately.
- digitization of the doctor's data and patient's data, including pathology reports and other related reports
- Another biggest challenge is to evaluate the trustworthiness of the doctor's data and patient's data stored in the Cloud. Further, elimination/blocking of the untrustworthiness records.

METHODOLOGY

The main aim of the proposed approach is to recognize the pneumonia symptoms in a child well before and identifying patients at risk of admission into hospitals. This approach will help the doctors in taking appropriate decisions for giving better treatment at right time. This approach proposed in this proposal will establish a system that can efficiently use resources and can potentially save millions lives and healthcare dollars each year.

Figure 1 shows the preliminary and broad framework of the proposed healthcare system. Several components of the proposed model and their expected contribution are discussed below.

This approach assumes that all the doctors, patients, staff and parents as stakeholders of the cloud and who will disseminate information through the cloud. The motive for considering cloud-based treatment for childhood pneumonia is its rapid

Figure 1. Layered architecture of proposed approach

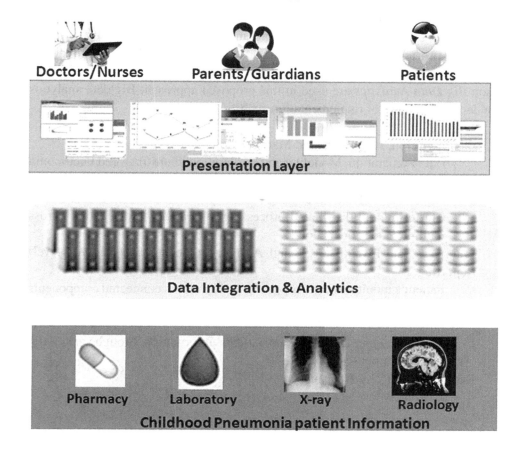

service provisioning and on-demand usage patterns. The in-patient's and out-patient's information gathered in each hospital is stored in cloud and inter connectivity of all the hospitals data is integrated through cloud. The data stored in cloud can be shared to all the stakeholders of the cloud across the globe. Further, the health data of all the diseases in particularly pneumonia patient's data is stored in cloud and can be used by any doctor across the globe at any time.

Due to this reason the proposed approach adopted cloud as a basis to store the childhood pneumonia patient's data. By doing in such a way any doctor can have access to this data for the best way to treat pneumonia. Doctors can also share their opinions and views by updating information in the cloud regarding the health conditions, abnormal behavior of child with pneumonia and any other relevant information which they feel mandatory for further use.

Cloud is having growing with the health information in the form of digitized scan reports, digitized X-Rays, and other pathology reports in it and the healthcare data is becoming *Big Data*. The data is of different kinds like structured and unstructured. Accessing unstructured vast variety of data and analyzing such big data requires efficient algorithms to acquire relevant data within short span of time. Due to this reason *Big Data Analytics* are used in this proposed approach. Big data analytics include several stages of implementation such as

- Data Ingestion, Integration and Manipulation
  - Data Preparation, Modeling and Exploration of unstructured Pneumonia Patients Data.
  - High Volume Data Processing
  - Clustering and distributed processing the patient's information across multiple nodes on a Cloud
- Enterprise (at Hospital level) and Ad-hoc (at parents and patients level) Reporting
  - Patient's monitoring and reporting to the various connected components like parents, doctors, nurses etc.
- Data Discovery and Visualization
  - Visual designer for processing patients' information through various development phases.
- Required Predictive Analysis
  - Extremely fast and readily decisive information

And, these phases will deploy a Big Data Analytics layer in the proposed model exclusively to address the pediatric Pneumonia specific patients' informatics.

Several analytics platforms will be adapted in the proposed approach including MapReducers like Hadoop, NoSQLs (for unstructured data) like Cassandra and MongoDB, SQLs (for structured data) like Informix, Ingres, Interbase, LucidDB, SQL Server, MySQL, Oracle, Postgres, Sybase and Teradat. Further, Powerful algorithms such as classification, regression, clustering and association will be used for predictive analysis and typical tools like Predictive Modeling Mark-up Language (PMML) will be used for visualizing the results and reports.

Treatment Steps

The proposed approach in this chapter will help the doctors in taking appropriate decisions in giving better treatment to child with pneumonia. This approach will provide decimated information present globally and gives expert doctors treatments as suggested treatment from the analytics taken from cloud storage. This proposed approach will help the doctors to give better treatment to childhood pneumonia outpatient as well as inpatient.

Outpatient

Whenever patient with pneumonia symptoms approaches the doctor as outpatient, doctor enquires about the symptoms like cough, cold, high temperature and headaches etc., A cloud-based application environment is provided to the doctor to enter the symptoms of patient, background medical history and any details related to previous admission into hospitals. Based on the details entered by the doctor, the application environment shows suggested treatments from cloud storage which is consolidated from all doctors treatment who treated the related patients with same medical background and symptoms. It also suggests the tests to be conducted for further examination and medical prescriptions of reputed doctors who treated the similar type of cases. And the suggestions are also showed to the doctor in highest rating suggestion to lowest rating suggestion. Based on the suggested solutions doctor can have a chance to choose the best and if required he can also contact the concerned doctor for further suggestions. So, cloud-based trustworthy servicing of treatment will help the doctor to choose best treatment from various suggested treatments. So that doctor will get best possible solutions on the fly to treat the patient effectively, efficiently and timely. Due to this approach the number of admissions into hospitals can be reduced by taking prompt decisions and timely treatment. Otherwise delay in identifying patients with pneumonia who are at high-risk will cause hospital admissions. This approach will reduce the healthcare cost as well as unnecessary admissions into hospitals by suggesting right decision at right time.

Inpatient

A patient with pneumonia is approaches the doctor very lately and he/she needs admission into hospital due to severity of disease. In general, whenever he admits into hospital as inpatient then a new case sheet is opened for him/her. This cloud-based trustworthy servicing is a novel approach where inpatient information is maintained in *digitized case sheets*. In this process, in-patient entries such as symptoms, treatment, diet and medicine information is updated in digitized case sheets by concerned doctors and staff. The information which is updated in the digitized case sheets are directly connected with cloud storage and updates which are made are stored in cloud storage. Whenever a doctor visits the patient then he may suggest some medicine, tests and diet etc., these entries are updated in the digitized case sheets by the doctor. The same is viewed by the staff nurses and after giving scheduled treatment, staff also updates the digitized case sheet by entering their treatment information.

If the patient needs any treatment from a consulting doctor, then the consulting doctor can check the details of the patient through online and he can also check the details of undergone treatment till date before he visits to the patient. If possible consulting doctor will directly suggest the treatment from his work place with the help of cloud-based treatment environment. All the data about the patient will be available to all the doctors who are giving treatment to the patient and even they know the treatment details which he has undergone in the process of inpatient through digitized case sheets.

The delays in getting the expert doctors from different places to visiting the patient are minimized due to this approach. Delay in giving right and timely treatment to children with pneumonia will cause sudden deaths. Giving best treatment is required in case of childhood pneumonia to reduced childhood deaths. This approach also reduces the cost of treatment by minimizing consulting doctor's efforts for traveling to visit the patient. Further this patient data can be used as a use case for other doctors because these all devices of different doctors are inter connected to cloud and all the entries are saved directly in the cloud storage. These entries may help the out-patient to avoid unnecessary admissions into hospitals.

Whenever a new patient approaches a doctor then patient will provide his previous history and symptoms, these are entered in specified application. Based on the entries given by doctor, this model maps the words in corresponding ontology database and different ontology retrieval algorithms are applied to identify relevant information. In this process, in every stage cloud-based trustworthy servicing model suggests the doctor by viewing suggested treatment according to the similar symptoms and based on the current health status of the patient. These suggestions are formed by applying big data analytics on different patient's data to come to a decision and gives appropriate information to the doctor by analyzing the patient's symptoms with cloud storage symptoms which are of similar type. While collecting the details from the big storage it will apply big data retrieval techniques to retrieve the relevant information. After getting this information it will apply the analytics on it to analyze the data to give possible suggestions given by different doctors.

The doctor's suggestions who gave treatment for the similar type of cases are displayed to the doctor who is giving treatment to the patient currently. The genuinity of doctor's suggestions are measured with trustworthy ratings. Every doctor is rated based on the feedbacks or recommendations made by different doctors who already taken their suggestions and succeeded to give best treatment and also the feedback given by patients. Every doctor has to undergo the evaluation process of finding trustworthiness of his suggestions. In this process, trust evaluation of each doctor's suggestion is done based on the direct impression achieved by the present doctor and indirect impression evaluated based the recommendations given by different doctors or patients about this doctor's treatment. So, based the trust values of the suggestions they are given rating. So, wherever a doctor enters the details of patient, he may be viewing suggested treatment by different doctors which is based on the rating of suggestion. That means best rated doctors suggestion is listed first in the list, subsequently lowest rated suggestion. So, the doctor can suggest best solution amongst possible solutions for giving better treatment for the patient in-time. Now, based the retrieved information with trustworthy rating, this information is provided to the doctor as suggested treatment. Different algorithms need to device for mining of data accurately and efficiently, identifying trustworthiness of data and big data analytics to be adopted to give relevant suggestions to the doctors to give timely treatment.

This automated information may help the doctor to deliver timely, effective treatment to pneumonia patients. This new way of approach will give accurate and cost effective treatment for childhood pneumonia by considering previous treatment history by collaborate with other doctors, at first point of interaction. This innovate treatment initiate will give assurance to all children by suggesting appropriate treatment and referral. With the use of proposed approach, childhood pneumonia deaths can be reduced.

Outcomes of The Proposed Approach

- A complete cloud-based childhood Pneumonia detection system using Cloud and Big Data Analytics
- A model Cloud-based storage system for pediatric Pneumonia patient's information and accessing
- Generalized Prototype healthcare system suitable for other diseases with minimal changes
- A Cloud computing system for providing services to other users.

Benefits of this Approach

1. Digitization of patient's data in *digitized case sheets* for storing patient's data in centralized storage i.e., cloud storage.
2. With digitized case sheets, reduction of paper work leading to cost cutting, no loss of data due to paper spoilage. And no need for a physical record room to maintain correspondences and files leading to major savings on physical storage space.
3. Patient's Diagnostic reports, X-ray and scanning reports etc., are stored in cloud storage.
4. Doctor's prescriptions, reports are also stored in cloud storage.
5. Genuinity of doctor's suggestions are measured with trustworthy ratings.

6. Patient's feedback about treatment is considered.
7. Suggested best doctors list with their opinions are displayed to doctor in fast and better treatment of pneumonia patients.
8. Big data analytics will provide accurate and faster results compared to manual diagnosis
9. Untrustworthy records may be blocked or eliminated. This way, accuracy levels of the data may be maintained.

CONCLUSION

This chapter proposes a new way of treatment to childhood pneumonia patients to save guard/ reduce the childhood deaths. This new way of approach will retrieve disseminated information from the cloud storage and analyze the data to give better suggestions to the doctors who are treating the childhood pneumonia patients. Due to interoperable, scalable and integrated IT infrastructure nature of cloud, this approach adopted cloud as a basis to store required information. The cloud will store patient's pathological reports, x-rays, blood test reports, doctor's prescriptions and various reports. In case of inpatient treatment, this approach uses digitized case sheets to store the information about the patient's diet, medicines and treatment details. By using these digitized case sheets reduction of usage of paper work, no loss of data due to paper spoilage. This approach will also consider genuinity of the doctors based on trustworthiness ratings. Big data analytics will provide accurate and faster results for better treatment. This chapter provides benefits of this approach and gives innovative treatment to save the child. The following things should be followed by the patients for their better life even after innovative technologies such as Big Data and Cloud provided to them which can give accurate and precise diagnosis. (1) Patients should live in right manner by following appropriate steps to improve their health condition (2) Appropriate care should be taken by patient by considering coordinated information from caregivers (3) Choosing the right professionals or doctors for his/her treatment by knowing the track records of professionals or doctors who give best outcomes in previous history. One should know the innovative approaches in the healthcare domain and can choose the appropriate one which gives the better diagnosis and right healthcare delivery. This proposal is coining to save the child from Pneumonia by designing and developing an effective, efficient and timely treatment mechanism using latest technologies such as Cloud and Big Data Analytics.

REFERENCES

Bottles, K., & Begoli, E. (2014). Understanding the pros and cons of big data analytics. *Physician Executive, 40,* 6–12. PMID:25188972

Chawla, N. V., & Davis, D. A. (2013). Bringing *big data to personalized healthcare: A patient-centered framework. Journal of General Internal Medicine, 28*(S3), S660–S665. doi:10.1007/s11606-013-2455-8 PMID:23797912

Chen, H. C., Chiang, R. H. L., & Storey, V. C. (2012). Business intelligence and analytics: From big data to big impact. *Management Information Systems Quarterly, 36,* 1165–1188.

Chorafas, D. (2011). *Cloud Computing Strategies.* Taylor and Francis Group, LLC.

Dillon, T., Wu, C., & Chang, E. (2010). Cloud Computing: Issues and Challenges. In *Proceedings of Advanced Information Networking and Applications (AINA), 2010 24th IEEE International Conference on.* doi:10.1201/9781439834541

Halamka, J. D. (2014). Early experiences with big data at an academic medical center. *Health Affairs, 33*(7), 1132–1138. doi:10.1377/hlthaff.2014.0031 PMID:25006138

Helm-Murtagh, S. C. (2014). Use of Big Data by Blue Cross and Blue Shield of North Carolina. *NCMJ, 75,* 195–197. PMID:24830494

Jennings, R. (2009). *Cloud Computing with the Windows Azure Platform.* Wrox Press Ltd.

Marks, E. (2008). *Service-Oriented Architecture (SOA) Governance for the Services Driven Enterprise.* Wiley.

Mccracken, G. H., Jr. (2000). Etiology and treatment of pneumonia. *Pediatric Infectious Disease Journal, 19*(4), 373-377.

Miller, K. (2012). Big data analytics in biomedical research. *Biomedical Computation Review.*

Pring, B. (2011). *Forecast: Public Cloud Services, Worldwide and Regions, Industry Sectors, 2010-2015, 2011 Update.* Gartner, Inc.

Rittinghouse, J., & Ransome, J. (2009). *Cloud Computing: Implementation, Management, and Security.* CRC Press, Inc.

Schultz, T. (2013). Turning healthcare challenges into big data opportunities: A use-case review across the pharmaceutical development lifecycle. *Bull. Association Inform. Sci. Technol., 39,* 34–40. doi:10.1002/bult.2013.1720390508

Terry, N. P. (2013). Protecting patient privacy in the age of big data. *UMKC Law Review, 81,* 385–415.

UNICEF. (2008). *Countdown to 2015. Tracking progress in maternal, neonatal and child survival: the 2008 report.* New York: UNICEF.

Vaquero, L., Rodero-Merino, L., Caceres, J., & Lindner, M. (2008). A break in the clouds: Towards a cloud definition. *SIGCOMM Comput. Commun. Rev., 39*(1), 50–55. doi:10.1145/1496091.1496100

Velte, A., Velte, T., & Elsenpeter, R. (2010). *Cloud Computing A Practical Approach.* McGraw-Hill.

Warner, D. (2013). *Safe de-identification of big data is critical to health care.* Health Inform. Manage.

White, S.E., (2014). A review of big data in health care: Challenges and opportunities. *Open Access Bio inform., 6,* 13-18. DOI: 10.2147/OAB.S50519

Yang, S., Njoku, M., & Mackenzie, C. F. (2014). 'Big data' approaches to trauma outcome prediction and autonomous resuscitation. *British Journal of Hospital Medicine, 75*(11), 637–641. doi:10.12968/hmed.2014.75.11.637 PMID:25383434

Chapter 6
Diabetes Patients Monitoring by Cloud Computing

Sepideh Poorejbari
Pervasive and Cloud Computing Laboratory, Iran

Hamed Vahdat-Nejad
University of Birjand, Iran

Wathiq Mansoor
University in Dubai, UAE

ABSTRACT

The healthcare system is important due to the focus on human care and the interference with human lives. In recent years, we have witnessed a rapid rise in e-healthcare technologies such as Electronic Health Records (EHR) and the importance of emergency detection and response. Cloud computing is one of the new approaches in distributed systems that can handle some of the challenges of smart healthcare in terms of security, sharing, integration and management. In this study, an architecture design of a cloud-based pervasive healthcare system for diabetes treatment has been proposed. For this, three different components are defined as follows: (1) The home context manager which gathers necessary information from patients while simultaneously providing feedback, (2) a patient health record manager that is accessible by nurses or physicians at the hospital, and (3) a diabetes management system which is located with the cloud infra-structure for managing and accessing patient's information. The performance of proposed architecture is demonstrated through a user scenario.

DOI: 10.4018/978-1-5225-1002-4.ch006

INTRODUCTION

Information technology can play a vital role in healthcare services in terms of electronic health. Recent advances in e-health can be broadly defined as the application of information and communication technologies in healthcare systems (Varshney, 2009). Making use of the internet for storing, accessing and modifying healthcare information and digitizing many processes and tasks is a necessary step for realizing e-health. In this case, we have the advantages of e-health such as a rise in the quality of services in aging societies, reduction in cost and in medical errors and the ease by which data can be moved to the right place. However, digitizing paper-based records, collecting and storing medical information as well as lack of suitable technology for preventive care can become rather challenging.

After the emergence of the pervasive computing paradigm, pervasive healthcare technology has been proposed to support a wide range of applications and services including patient monitoring and emergency response. However, they simultaneously introduce several challenges including data storage and management, interoperability, availability of resources and ubiquitous access issues (Ziefle & Rocker, 2010).

Diabetes is one of the major chronic diseases in the world. Diabetes, often referred to by doctors as diabetes mellitus, describes a group of metabolic diseases in which the person has high blood glucose (blood sugar), either because insulin production is inadequate, or because the body's cells do not respond properly to insulin, or both. Diabetes manifests itself in three types:

Type 1: This type of diabetes is usually diagnosed in children and young adults, and was previously known as juvenile diabetes. Only 5% of people with diabetes have this form of the disease. In this type of diabetes, the body does not produce insulin.

Type 2: Is a problem with your body that causes blood glucose (sugar) levels to rise higher than normal. This is also called hyperglycemia. Type 2 is the most common form of diabetes; About 90 percent of people with diabetes have type 2 diabetes.

Type 3: Gestational Diabetes is a temporary condition that occurs during pregnancy. It affects approximately 2 to 4 percent of all pregnancies and involves an increased risk of developing diabetes for both the mother and child.

All forms of diabetes increase a patient's risk of emerging different health complications. Short-term complications such as hypoglycemia and hyperglycemia (very low and high blood glucose), and long-term complications such as eyes, heart, kidneys, nerves and feet failure are serious and life-threatening. The proper management of blood glucose levels reduces the risk of developing these complications. Factors such as the illness that patient suffers, treatment, physical and psychological stress, physical activity, drugs and diet (meal plan) can cause unpredictable and dangerous consequences such as hypoglycemia, hyperglycemia, and falling into a coma.

The management of diabetes is becoming an increasingly important problem worldwide. In 2014, according to the International Diabetes Federation, at least 387 million people (or 8.3% world population) suffered from diabetes and it is expected that by 2035, the number of diabetes will increase to more than 590 million.

Case Study: This scenario originates from the Imam Reza hospital, one of the leading and technical hospitals in Mashhad, Iran.
Mr. Toosi, a 62 year old man has suffered from type 2 diabetes for more than 10 years. In this period of time, he has caught different health complications such as diabetes foot, eye problems, high blood pressure, and heart problems. His prescription includes 20 units of insulin per day, 12 units in the morning and 8 units at night. In addition he has to check his glucose level on a daily basis. On one early morning, Mr. Toosi woke up with shortness of breath and weakness in his body. Without special attention, he had his breakfast and injects his insulin. After two hours he feels more pain and weakness in his chest and body, but because he is alone at home he prefers to wait until one of the family members returns home, before heading out for a check-up. When Mr Toosi's son arrives home, he immediately drives his father to the nearest hospital. At the hospital, the physicians and nurses run some treatments, however due to the lack of medical information and patient health records they are unable to make precise decisions and prefer to send the patient to the hospital where Mr. Toosi's main physician is available. Unfortunately, after sending the patient to another hospital he falls into a diabetes coma and passes away after a second heart attack.

The above scenario leads to a few issues that need to be addressed in pervasive diabetes health system. Here we focus on the following two problems:

- Monitoring patient remotely at home and detecting and managing different situations.
- Accessing patient health records and medical history at anytime and anywhere by legal persons.

The concept of cloud-based pervasive healthcare system is a new paradigm for the healthcare sector that uses cloud computing to treat, manage and control patients pervasively. The systems are supported by different algorithms, cloud infrastructures, smart homes, devices, and sensors and create several service types according to their context and environment. This paper presents a Cloud-based pervasive healthcare system architecture for treating diabetes, in order to manage and control diabetic patients and reduce the hypoglycemia and hyperglycemia conditions and consequently their risks. The system, which we will refer to as DICPer-Health, is designed to control patients pervasively at their homes. Three environments including a home, hospital and cloud structure are considered as main parts of this system, by which each of these sections has its own components and acts separately.

We have selected diabetes type 2 as the chronic condition cannot be cured and is the condition of 9/10 diabetes patients. In type 2 diabetes, the body cannot use insulin properly. This is called insulin resistance. Type 2 is treated with lifestyle changes, oral medications, and insulin injections. This type of diabetes usually gets worse over time, and in order for individuals with type 2 diabetes to control their blood glucose levels, they need to eat healthy, stay active, and use prescribed drugs appropriately. In this case we have considered three important factors in our framework; diet, activity, and insulin. These three factors control and manage the lifestyle of type 2 diabetes patients.

The following sections of the paper are organized as follows; Section (2) presents the pervasive healthcare projects and related works. Section (3) presents architecture to support diabetes treatment. The architecture parts are described in subsections. Section (4) presents the evaluation of work according to real life patient scenario. Finally, section 5 will conclude the paper.

RELATED WORKS

Today, there is a great amount of research work in the field of pervasive healthcare to improve e-health services; however only a few number target the use of cloud infrastructure as a new IT paradigm and are surveyed as below.

"The Integrated Cloud-based Healthcare Infrastructure" project, ICHI has been developed in Edinburgh Napier University of United Kingdom. ICHI presents a system that integrates a formal care system (DACAR) with an informal care system (Microsoft Health Vault) that enables not only sharing and access of health records right along the patient pathway, but also provides a high level of security and privacy within a cloud environment (Ekonomou, Fan, Buchanan, & Thuemmler, 2011). Another project in the University of Central Greece, "Bringing IoT and Cloud Computing towards Pervasive Healthcare", IoTC, proposes a platform based on cloud computing for management of mobile and wearable healthcare sensors (Mu-Hsing Kuo, 2011). In another research project concluded at the University of Greece, namely "Managing Wearable Sensor Data through Cloud Computing" (MWSC), a wearable textile platform that collects motion and heartbeat data and stores them wirelessly on an open cloud infrastructure for monitoring and further processing was studied (Wan, Zou, Ullah, Lai, Zhou & Wang, 2013). "Cloud-Enabled Wireless Body Area Networks for Pervasive Healthcare (CWBAN)" is another article in the same context that focuses on a cloud-enabled WBAN architecture and its applications are within pervasive healthcare systems. CWBAN develops WBANs with MCC (Mobile Cloud Computing) capability, a Cloud-Enabled WBAN (Woon Ahn, Cheng, Baek, Jo & Chen, 2013). This project has also been developed in different universities including South China University of Technology, King Saud University, and the University of British Columbia. Another article namely "An Auto-Scaling Mechanism for Virtual Resources to Support Mobile, Pervasive, and Real-Time Healthcare Applications in Cloud Computing" (RTHA) proposes a novel server-side auto-scaling mechanism. The model is based on cloud computing with virtualization technologies in collaboration with the University of Houston and Korea University (Corredor, Tarrio, Bernardos, & Casar, 2013).

As mentioned above, the number of pervasive healthcare projects related to cloud computing for diabetes are few. Moving forward, we have scrutinized just two articles that introduce a personal health system (PHS) to manage diabetic patients. One of these projects at the University of London, is "COMMODITY$_{12}$: A Smart e-Health Environment for Diabetes Management" that emphasizes on designing the PHS to address major problems of both diabetic patients and doctors who treat diabetes (Kafah et al., 2013). COMMODITY$_{12}$ consists of ambient, wearable and portable devices, which acquire, monitor and communicate physiological parameters and other health factors and vital body signals of a patient. In this system, there are intelligent agents that use expert biomedical knowledge to interpret data and then present a feedback from a patient's health status directly to the patient from the device (Kafah et al., 2013).

University of Murcia, Spain, has developed another healthcare project for diabetes, "An Internet of Things-based Personal device for Diabetes Therapy Management in Ambient Assisted Living (AAL)", that presents a personal diabetes management device based on the Internet of Things. The target is to support a patient's insulin therapy to decrease hyperglycemia and hypoglycemia counts and the risks involved (Jara, Zamora, & Skarmeta, 2011). This project focuses more on insulin dosage based on mobile assistance services. The project considers different factors such as the illness that patients suffer, drugs, treatments, stress, physical activity and meal (diet) for insulin therapy.

One related survey is "An Introduction to Cloud-Based Pervasive Healthcare Systems", that reviews different projects in healthcare sector with the focus on cloud computing (Poorejbari & Vahdat-nejad, 2014).

THE PROPOSED FRAMEWORK

Overview

To introduce DICPer-Health, our first initiative is to present the general architecture of the system in order to briefly describe the main components. We will then concentrate on the description of three key components: Home Context Manager, Hospital Environment and Cloud Infrastructure.

Figure 1 depicts our proposed architecture for a smart healthcare environment. The figure consists of three main components which are connected via Internet: (i) The home context manager which gathers necessary information from patients while simultaneously providing feedback, (ii) a patient health record form that is accessible by nurses or physicians at the hospital, and (iii) a diabetes management system which is located with the cloud infrastructure for managing and accessing patient's information.

In our proposed architecture, the home context manager plays a major role in collecting, storing and processing data. Once the initial procedures are complete,

Figure 1. General Architecture of DICPer-Health

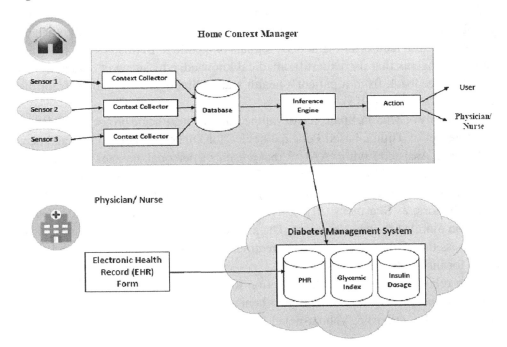

the system presents alerts, suitable treatments, and advices to the patient. The function of the home context manager and its components will be described in a later section.

Home Context Manager

The main role of the home context manager is collecting different information such as blood glucose level, blood pressure, and heart rates from patients through various sensors at specific times. After gathering patient health parameters, all the required information is stored in a context database. The inference engine then infers two different important conditions; High risk and emergency situations. According to the conditions and patient health history, suitable advices and alarms will be communicated to the patient's smart device or in an application connected to nurses or experts. The home context manager consists of the following components.

Wireless Sensors

Sensors are essential components in smart environments which sense and collect physical parameters. We utilize three types of wireless sensors in our framework, which gather fundamental physiological information from diabetes. The sensors are depicted in Table 1 and described below with the objective of sensing our requirements.

- Glucose monitoring by finger prick (GlucoTel Sensor).
- Blood pressure monitoring (PressureTel Sensor)
- Heart rate monitoring (Pulse Sensor)

None of the above sensors are expected to be considered obtrusive by the patients. Patients without any special knowledge can use them with ease.

Table 1. Schema of context table

Parameter	Date	Time			
		8 A.M.	10 A.M.	3 P.M.	10 P.M.
Blood Glucose					
Blood Pressure					
Heart Rate					

Context Collector

After sensing raw data by sensors, the context collector collects the data and delivers the information to the context database. 6LoWPAN is a technology for transferring sensed data to smart devices. This technology connects wireless clinical devices like glucometer to the smart environments or gateways. We proposed 6LoWPAN technology for sending data from the sensors to the context collectors and then by using SQL statements, context collector inserts data into the context database.

Context Database

This database consists of one table, namely the context table by which physiological parameters are the defined fields (Table 1).

The parameter field is designed to evaluate a patients important physiological factors such as blood glucose, blood pressure, and heart rate levels. The date and time fields reveal patient check-up timings. For diabetic patients monitoring and managing blood glucose is an essential task as blood glucose levels should remain within normal ranges. There are two types of blood glucose measures that are very important in a diabetic treatment; FBS[1] and the THG[2] level check-up. In this case we have proposed four specific times in order to measure these parameters. It begins early morning at 8 A.M. for an initial measuring FBS, 10 A.M. for measuring the 2 hours glucose level after breakfast meal, 3 P.M. for evaluating the 2 hours glucose level after lunch time, and 10 P.M. for evaluating the 2 hours glucose level after dinner. In addition the patient's blood pressure and heart rate levels will be checked simultaneously. After monitoring all the parameters via wireless sensors, the sensed data will be stored in a context table, by which the inference engine can use them for inferring suitable outcomes.

Inference Engine

The inference engine determines two principal situations; high risk and emergency based upon specified rules and algorithms. The inputs of the inference engine are the context table data and, the outputs of this function in high risk condition, is a patient form that shows alarms and useful advices such as practical diet, activity and correct insulin dosage, and in emergency situation, is a nurse or physician form that presents an alarm and dangerous factors to the nurse or experts.

In our proposed framework, the data interpretation is based on the specific rules and defaults. Moving forward, we will describe the basic definitions and default rules.

Table 2. Glucose different ranges

	Very Low	**Low**	**Normal**	**High**	**Very High**
Glucose Level	<70	70-90	90-126	120-200	200<

Table 2 presents the normal and abnormal range of blood glucose levels and the unit of blood glucose is measured as mg/dl (milligrams per deciliter). And all physicians and experts try to keep the patient blood glucose level at the normal range.

So, the rules of our proposed architecture are defined according to these ranges for distinguishing hypoglycemia and hyperglycemia conditions.

The other important parameter is the blood pressure levels that should be considered. Most diabetic patients have a high blood pressure problem that requires monitoring. The normal range of blood pressure is between 80-120 mmHg (millimeter of mercury), ranges are considered abnormal when reaching the upper range at approximately 135 mmHg. If the blood pressure of a patient becomes more than 135 mmHg, then the system recommends some treatments for this condition.

Heart rate is another essential factor in diabetes treatment. The normal range of a heart pulse is 60-100 beats per minute (bpm). In our system, we have labeled it as "Low", if the number of the heart rate becomes less than 50 bpm, and "High" if the number of the heart pulse reaches more than 100 bpm.

Diet and meals play an essential role in diabetes treatment and control of blood glucose level. According to nutritional views, diabetes patients are required to have a specific amount of nutrients such as carbohydrate, fiber, sodium and protein in their daily meals. The proposed amounts of nutrients are classified in Table 3.

For daily activities, the body needs energy and this energy comes from foods. Each food has a specific amount of calories. The number of calories the body consumes in a day is different for every individual.

In our proposed framework, according to the calculated energy for each patient, the amount of carbohydrate that should be used by patients is at least 55 percent and at most 70 percent of a patient total energy. The amount of fiber is 20-30 grams,

Table 3. Range of nutrients in daily meals

Carbohydrate	**Fiber**	**Sodium**	**Protein**
55%- 70%	20-35 gr	2000-3000 mg	15%-20%

the amount of sodium is 2000-3000 milligrams and the range of protein is 15 to 20 percent of total daily calories.

The inference engine interprets acquired data according to various rules that we have described, and grouped into five rules in the following sections.

First, 2 different emergency situations are described in Case 1 and Case 2. And to continue 3 high-risk conditions are shown.

Case 1:

```
If (FBS is very high and PR is low and BP is high) or
     (THG is very high and PR is low and BP is high)
          Then
               Emergency Situation;
```

Case 1 shows a condition where FBS or THG is very high and simultaneously the pulse rate is low and blood pressure is high. In this case we have labeled this condition as 'Emergency Situation', meaning fast and critical treatments are required.

Case 2:

```
If (FBS is very low and PR is high) or
     (THG is very low and PR is high) then
          Emergency Situation;
```

In Case 2, when the fasting blood sugar level is very low and the pulse rate is high, or when the two hours glucose level is very low and the pulse rate is high, then it is immediately labeled as an emergency situation. In this case the inference engine sends an alert to the nurses or physicians. As a result medical professionals become aware of the critical situation, allowing the experts to act immediately.

Case 3:

```
If (FBS is low and PR is high) or
     (THG is low and PR is high) then
          Diet:
               (Use 15gr carb)
               (Carbohydrate is high)
               (Protein is high)
               If (BP is high) then (Sodium is low)
                    Else (Sodium is medium)
          Activity:
               Stop for at least 15 min.
```

```
Insulin:
        Increase 2-unit insulin dosage
```

Case 3 presents a condition where the FBS of a patient is low and the pulse rate is high, or the THG is low and PR is high. In this case suitable treatments related to the diet appear in the patient smart device. As a result the patient is notified that he/she should eat 15 grams of carbohydrates immediately in order to prevent hypoglycemia. The amount of carbohydrate and protein can be maximum for the other meals. There is a rule here, if the patient blood pressure is high then the amount of sodium must be at a minimum level, otherwise it is average. In this scenario, the patient must stop activity for at least 15 minutes. Insulin dosage can increase 2 units.

Case 4:

```
If (FBS is very high and PR is low) or
      (THG is very high and PR is low) then
            Diet:
                      (Carbohydrate is low)
                      (Protein is low)
                      (Fiber is high)
                      (Sodium is low)
            Activity:
                  Stop for at least 15 min.
```

Another high-risk condition is presented in case 4. In this case the FBS or THG is very high and PR is low, so for diet the amount of carbohydrate, protein, and sodium is low and the amount of fiber is high. With regards to patient activity, it is suggested that the patient does not perform any kind of sport or other related activities for the next 15 minutes. The patient may decrease 2 unit of insulin dosage for better control and treatment.

When the FBS and THG levels are high then a diet is proposed where by the amount of carbohydrate and sodium are maintained at a minimum level, and the fiber levels remain high. In this condition, if there is a kidney problem the amount of protein should be low.

Case 5:

```
If (FBS is high) or (THG is high) then
            Diet:
                      (Carbohydrate is low)
                      If there is a kidney problem then
                                  (Protein is low)
```

```
                    (Fiber is high)
                    (Sodium is low)
        Activity:
            Walking for 15 min.
```

Case 5 shows another high-risk condition where FBS or THG is high. In this condition carbohydrates should be kept at a low level and again the kidney problem should be considered. For fiber, it's high in daily meals and sodium is low. It is suggested that walking for 15 minutes can help to control the glucose level.

Hospital Environment

Before a patient can be monitored and treated in a smart home environment, medical experts are required to collect important and useful clinical information prior to initiation. All the health information related to diabetes will be gathered in a hospital environment. In our proposed work, we have designed a patient health record form that should be completed by a nurse or physician. A complete compilation of data including diabetes tests, health history, and insulin dosage information will be stored in a table, called the patient health record (PHR) The PHR is centralized within the cloud infrastructure in order to provide the health information necessary for detection alerts and treatments according to the medical professional analysis. In the next section we will look at the cloud structure.

Cloud Structure

The use of the cloud has provided many benefits to the proposed structure such accessibility, flexibility, globalizing, reducing costs and so on. The main goal of using cloud computing in our framework is, designing a diabetes management system in cloud structure that can be accessible at anytime, anywhere. We have proposed a public cloud like the GoogleAppEngine as a cloud infrastructure. In this case the diabetes management system consists of three databases that are described in following subsections.

PHR Table

This table consists of patient health information that are gathered by nurses or physicians. The PHR table includes three types of information; Personal information (Table 4), Tests information (Table 5) and the history of different diseases and problems (Table 6).

Table 4. Patient personal information

P-ID	Name/ Family	Birth Date	Height	Weight	Address

Table 5. Patient medical tests

HbA1C	FBS	GTT	UG	Keton	Chol

Table 6. Patient problems

Heart	Kidney	Blood pressure	Surgery

GI Table

Glycemic Index is a number associated with a particular type of food that indicates the food's effect on a person's blood glucose. Foods with low glycemic index and glycemic load are suitable for diabetes. The inference engine with use of the information retrieved from the GI table, advice may be provided regarding appropriate foods in diabetes meals.

ID3 Table

The insulin dosage table consists of all insulin information related to a patient. Information such as insulin dosage, insulin types, and insulin units can be provided for every meal as shown in Table 8. All required data are gathered by professionals for better cure and treat.

Table 7. Glycemic index for different food

Food	GI	Serve (gr)	Carbohydrate	GL

Table 8. Patient insulin information

P-ID	Total Insulin	Insulin Units			Insulin Type	FBS	THG
		Morning	Noon	Night			

SCENARIO ANALYSIS

Based on the cloud-based pervasive healthcare framework we present, in this section, we analyze how it support the scenario described in the introduction. The whole operation process is illustrated by a UML sequence diagram shown in Figure 2.

When Mr. Toosi feels weakness and shortness of breath in the morning, according to our proposed framework he can measure his blood glucose, blood pressure and heart rate levels. According to the measured data, the proposed framework (home context manager) reveals the high risk factors, appropriate solutions and treatments in the patient's smart device. Under this scenario, Mr. Toosi is able to retrieve important information about his current condition, discover a treatment plan, and he may also ask for additional advice from his doctor about decreasing the high risk factors. In another condition where the family members decided to transfer their father to a hospital, the issue on arrival to the nearest hospital was the lack of information on Mr Toosi's condition. In this scenario all of Mr. Toosi's medical information will have already been stored in a diabetes management system. As a result, the information on the cloud will be accessible for physicians in emergency situations in order to support medical decisions.

Figure 2. Sequence diagram of framework

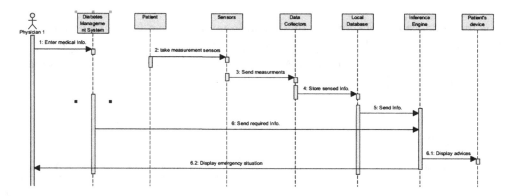

CONCLUSION

We have presented a structure supported by a cloud-based pervasive healthcare system that assists in controlling and managing diabetic patients. The aim is to empower their lifestyle and quality of life. The framework consists of different sensors, home context manager, hospital environment and cloud structures which acquire, monitor and process parameters. The data is interpreted by an inference engine that uses expert knowledge to derive important insights about the individual's health status. The data is presented as a feedback to the patient's smart device or physician portal.

Our work has focused on two important conditions, high risk and emergency situations and with the aim of reducing hypoglycemia and hyperglycemia conditions.

REFERENCES

Abowd, G. D., Dey, A. K., Brown, P. J., Davies, N., Smith, M., & Steggles, P. (1999). Towards a better understanding of context and context-awareness. In *1st International Symposium on Handheld and Ubiquitous Computing*. doi:10.1007/3-540-48157-5_29

Alicja Muras, J., Cahill, V., & Katherine Stokes, E. (2006). A taxonomy of pervasive healthcare systems. In Pervasive Health Conference and Workshops.

Bali, R., Troshani, I., & Wickramasinghe, N. (2013). *Pervasive Health Knowledge Management*. Springer. doi:10.1007/978-1-4614-4514-2

Bamiah, M., Brohi, S., & Chuprat, S. (2012). A study on significance of adopting cloud computing paradigm in healthcare sector. In *International Conference on Cloud Computing, Technologies, Applications & Management*. doi:10.1109/ICCCTAM.2012.6488073

Coronato, A., De Pietro, G., & Sannino, G. (2010). Middleware services for pervasive monitoring elderly and ill people in smart environments. In *Seventh International Conference on Information Technology*. doi:10.1109/ITNG.2010.139

Corredor, I., Tarrio, P., Bernardos, A. M., & Casar, J. R. (2013). An open architecture to enhance pervasiveness and mobility of health care services. *Communications in Computer and Information Science, 413*, 296–307. doi:10.1007/978-3-319-04406-4_30

Dooley, J. (2012). *Intelligent Environments Group*. University of Essex. Retrieved 6 18, 2014, from http://iieg.essex.ac.uk/idorm.htm/

Doukas, C., & Maglogiannis, I. (2011). Managing wearable sensor data through cloud computing. In *International Conference on Cloud Computing Technology and Science*. doi:10.1109/CloudCom.2011.65

Doukas, C., & Maglogiannis, I. (2012). Bringing IoT and cloud computing towards pervasive healthcare. In Innovative Mobile and Internet Services in Ubiquitous Computing. doi:10.1109/IMIS.2012.26

Ekonomou, M., Fan, L., Buchanan, W., & Thuemmler, C. (2011). An Integerated Cloud-based Healthcare Infrastructure. In *Third IEEE International Conference on Cloud Computing Technology and Science*. doi:10.1109/CloudCom.2011.80

Guo, B., Sun, L., & Zhang, D. (2010). The Architecture Design of a Cross-Domain Context Management System. In *8th IEEE international conference on pervasive computing and communications workshops*. doi:10.1109/PERCOMW.2010.5470618

Imam Reza Specialized & Sub-Specialized Hospital. (n.d.). Retrieved 3 05, 2014, from http://www.imamreza.ajaums.ac.ir

Jara, A. J., Zamora, M. A., & Skarmeta, A. F. G. (2011). An Internet of things-based personal device for diabetes therapy management in ambient assisted living (AAL). *Personal and Ubiquitous Computing*, *15*(4), 431–440. doi:10.1007/s00779-010-0353-1

Kafah, O., Bromuri, S., Sindlar, M., Weide, T., Aguilar Pelaez, E., Schaetchle, U., … Stathis, K. (2013). COMMODITY12: A smart e-health environment for diabetes management. *Journal of Ambient Intelligence and Smart Environments,* 479-502.

Le Bellego, G., Noury, N., Virone, G., Mousseau, M., & Demongeot, J. (2006). A model for the measurement of patient activity in a hospital suite. *Information Technology in Biomedicine,* 92-99.

Mell, P., & Grance, T. (2011). *NIST*. U.S Department of Commerce. Retrieved June 15, 2015 from http://www.nist.gov/itl/csd/cloud-102511.cfm

Mileo, A., Merico, D., & Bisiani, R. (2010). Support for context-aware monitoring in home healthcare. *Journal of Ambient Intelligence and Smart Environments,* 49-66.

Mu-Hsing Kuo, A. (2011). Opportunities and challenges of cloud computing to improve health care services. *Journal of Medical Internet Research*. PMID:21937354

Pardamean, B., & Rumanda, R. (2011). Integrated model of cloud-based e-medical record for health care organization. In *10th WSEAS International Conference on E-Activities*.

Poorejbari, S., & Vahdat-nejad, H. (2014). An Introduction to Cloud-Based Pervasive Healthcare Systems. In *4th international workshop on pervasive and context-aware middleware (PerCAM 14)*. doi:10.4108/icst.iccasa.2014.257442

Rantz, M., Skubic, M., Koopman, R., Phillips, L., Alexander, G., Miller, S., & Guevara, R. (2011). Using sensor networks to detect urinary tract infections in older adults. In *13th International Conference on e-Health Networking, Application and Services*. doi:10.1109/HEALTH.2011.6026731

Rashidi, P., & Cook, D. J. (2009). Keeping the Resident in the Loop: Adapting the Smart Home to the User. *IEEE Transactions on Systems, Man, and Cybernetics. Part A, Systems and Humans, 39*(5), 949–959. doi:10.1109/TSMCA.2009.2025137

Rashidi, P., & Mihailidis, A. (2013). A survey on ambient-assisted living tools for older adults. *IEEE Journal of Biomedical and Health Informatics, 17*(3), 579-590.

Shadab Ansari, W., Alamri, A. M., Hassan, M., & Shoaib, M. (2013). A survey on sensor-cloud: Architecture, Applications and Approaches. *International Journal of Distributed Sensor Networks*.

Singh, S., Puradkar, S., & Lee, Y. (2006). Ubiquitous Computing: Connecting Pervasive Computing through Semantic web. *Information Systems and e-Business Management, 4*(4), 421-439.

Tamura, T., Kawarada, A., Nambu, M., Tsukada, A., Sasaki, K., & Yamakoshi, K. I. (2007). E-healthcare at an experimental welfare techno house in Japan. *Open Medical Informatics*, 1-7.

Vahdat-nejad, H., Zamanifar, K., & Nematbakhsh, N. (2013). Context-aware middleware architecture for smart home environment. *International Journal of Smart Home, 7*, 77-86.

Varshney, U. (2009). *Pervasive Healthcare Computing: EMR/EHR*. Wireless and Health Monitoring. doi:10.1007/978-1-4419-0215-3

Wan, J., Zou, C., Ullah, S., Lai, C., Zhou, M., & Wang, X. (2013). Cloud-Enabled wireless body area networks for pervasive healthcare. *IEEE Network, 27*(5), 56–61. doi:10.1109/MNET.2013.6616116

Woon Ahn, Y., Cheng, A. M. K., Baek, J., Jo, M., & Chen, H. (2013). An auto-scaling mechanism for virtual resources to support mobile, pervasive, real-time health-care applications in cloud computing. *IEEE Network, 27*(5), 62–68. doi:10.1109/ MNET.2013.6616117

Zhang, R., Lee, M., & Liu, L. (2010). Security models and requirements for health-care application clouds. In *3rd International Conference on Cloud Computing*. doi:10.1109/CLOUD.2010.62

Zhang, Y., Lee, M., & Gatton, T. M. (2009). Agent-Based Healthcare Systems for Real-Time Chronic Diseases. In *2009 World Conference on Services-I*. doi:10.1109/SERVICES-I.2009.104

Ziefle, M., & Rocker, C. (2010). Acceptance of pervasive healthcare systems: A Comparison of Different Implementation Concepts. In *4th international conference on pervasive computing*. doi:10.4108/ICST.PERVASIVEHEALTH2010.8915

ENDNOTES

[1]   Fasting Blood Sugar
[2]   Two Hour Glucose
[3]   Insulin Dosage

Chapter 7
IBM's Watson Analytics for Health Care:
A Miracle Made True

Mayank Aggarwal
GKV, India

Mani Madhukar
IBM, India

ABSTRACT

With the advent of Internet and Computers, Information Technology (IT) has become a major tool to aid medical issues. IBM Watson is one such initiative by IBM, which provides integration with any application to build Internet of Things (IoT), based health applications and also assists by its existing services. The strength of Watson is its data analytics and Artificial Intelligence. The four variants of Watsons are Watson Discovery Advisor, Oncology, Clinical Trial Matching and Curam. It is based on Open Source Apache UIMA, Apache Lucene. Its integration with IBM Bluemix Cloud, Platform as a Service (PaaS) makes it easily available to users.

DOI: 10.4018/978-1-5225-1002-4.ch007

INTRODUCTION

The use of IT for health care is no longer a new concept. Use of computers and IT in every filed has become a common practice. Recording of patient histories, details, billing and other information in computers has become a common practice everywhere.

But the actual use needed is still missing in India.

According to an expert "75% of treatment are done on Trial Basis with not exact dosage of medicines and actual number of tests prescribed" such things result in millions of deaths per year in India. If we can have a collection of all records of patient histories countrywide and some way to predict on this basis it would be miracle.

IBM's Watson is one such miracle.

HISTORY

In 2011, in a TV show "Jeopardy" IBM's Watson defeated the Jeopardy's champion Ken Jennings and Brad Rutter. This gave birth to IBM's super computer Watson called after its founder Thomas J Watson (Best, 2011).

When the duel was finished, Watson had $77,147 resulting in loss of $21,600 and $24,000 to Rutter and Jennings respectively.

This was the victory of a machine over two humans and a birth of Artificial Intelligence with learning capacity in real sense.

David Ferrucci, principal investigator of Watson DeepQA technology, said Watson could conduct self-assessments and learn.

JOURNEY TOWARDS MEDICAL SCIENCE

The Jeopardy game was over but IBMers were not out to rest. The mission to make it the best doctor in world continued. This gave birth to IBM Watson Health Cloud. The team added the required information, checked for the results and modified it to give the best performance. Thousands of questions were asked and results checked if anything went wrong then it was corrected afterwards answers were given for which Watson has to ask the questions. Machine Learning enables questioning and answering model and also algorithms can be modified for better results.

In 2013 Watson used many textbooks, like PubMed and Medline and large number of records of different patients from Memorial Sloan Kettering. According to Forbes, 2013 605,000 medical symptoms, 25,000 training cases, 2 million notes have been analyzed and assistance of 14,700 clinician hours for its accuracy in generating the hypothesis.

IBM Watson Health Cloud for Life Sciences Compliance and IBM Watson Care Manager was launched in 2015. It has mergers with Columbia University, Boston Children's Hospital, ICON plc, Teva Pharmaceuticals and Sage Bionetworks

In 2015 acquisition of Merge Healthcare Inc. a leading company helping doctors to store and access medical images, gives a major breakthrough for Watson Health Cloud (Macmillan & Dowskin, 2015).

Important organizations in health-care already working with IBM Watson are Mayo Clinic, Memorial Sloan Kettering Cancer Center, Cleveland Clinic, New York Genome Center and the University of Texas MD Anderson Cancer Center. It has recently made its foray into Indian Medical scene.

Manipal Hospitals' have adopted Watson for Oncology, a cognitive computing platform trained by Memorial Sloan-Kettering Cancer Center, which uses records to give symptoms, based treatment options, it enables the doctors to give personalized attention to cancer patients on individual basis (Debroha, 2015).

The IBM Watson Health Cloud for Life Sciences Compliance can make medical science to do innovations in much simple and effective way, also deploy GxP compliant infrastructure keeping security, regulation of data in mind.

IBM Watson Care Manager is a population health solution that uniquely combines features of Apple's Health-Kit, Watson Health and Research-Kit, which enables iPhone users to study and research. It allows doctors to generate a broad range of determinants as per their patient's data to have good knowledge of the treatment and its outcome.

IN DEPTH

Watson is the pioneer to provide cognitive computing capability system available commercially giving rise to new era. The system uses cloud computing, collects high volume of data, analyze it, understands complicated and difficult questions asked in natural language, and gives proof based results.

At first system is told about the symptoms to the system, details like family history, undergoing treatment, duration of illness etc. are undertaken and analyzed. Using this information along with the findings from tests along with different types of treatment guidelines, digital record of medical cases and prescriptions of physicians, as well as peer-reviewed research and clinical studies. Then, Watson can gives different options for treatment and its confidence rating for each option. It uses the power of unstructured data (Feldman & Hanover, 2012).

Variants

Currently Watson Health Cloud provides various variants for different purposes as follow:

1. Watson Discovery Advisor for Life Sciences: It makes solutions easier by connecting and drawing relationships between different data sources so it can find something new.
2. Watson for Oncology: Trained by Memorial Sloan Kettering (MSK) it collaborates the patient's medical report with huge database along with current expert training from MSK physicians, histories of other cancer cases and more, which results in evidence based treatment options?
3. Watson for Clinical Trial Matching: It facilitates doctors to reduce all possible cancer trials and faster matching of appropriate trials, resulting in better and new treatment options for the patients.
4. Curam: By designing around the client, Cúram solutions empower organizations to collaborate around client needs and offer more effective ways to achieve desired health and social goals

Working of Watson

So the first question arises is how does Watson work and its use in health-care.

Watson makes use of Natural Language capabilities; Hypothesis generation and finally evidence based learning to learn from literature and case studies available. It then helps medical professionals in making their decision.

Watson can now assist a surgeon in diagnosing a disease or making subscription of medicines/surgery to the patient based on various parameters it takes into account while making the suggestion.

The process of getting a Watson recommendation for health-care professional can be explained in the following steps for more clarity:

1. It starts with the medical professional putting a question to the Watson system giving details of the symptoms and other relevant information that can make an impact.
2. Watson system starts parsing the inputs provided to identify important details. Watson has acquired skills on understanding medical terms and has Natural Language processing capabilities.
3. Watson mines the data of the patient to identify relevant information about the family of the patient, current treatments undertaken and other relevant data about the patient.

4. As a next step Watson, puts this information in a perspective to form Hypothesis, putting together information from patient history, medical tests etc.
5. Watson has capabilities to integrate electronic medical records of the patient, clinical studies, medical publications, guidelines for prognosis etc. with the patient data and analyze them together in one perspective gaining insights from the latest medical findings and how they can be useful in patient's diagnosis.

Armed with all the information, Watson now creates a list of potential diagnosis's mapping each with the information it had collected and collaborated. Each line item in the list of potential diagnosis has a score, which indicates the correctness of hypothesis.

This ability to gather all the related information and generate scores during the hypothesis generation makes Watson useful to solve the complex problems, also assists doctors to make accurate decisions and well informed.

The Watson engine workflow for analyzing the interpretation process of Watson can be explained with the help of Figure 1. The workflow explains the various stages that Watson undergoes to interpret, reason and find answers to any query being analyzed by Watson.

1. It generates a search query after parsing natural language question.
2. It gives all related information notes by its inbuilt search engine searching the vast amount of records.
3. It generates appropriate results (the hypotheses) by parsing the natural language based search results.
    a. In support of the generated hypothesis it collects evidences by constructing and initiating another search.
    b. Evidence to support each hypothesis is searched by inbuilt search engine.
    c. Evidences searched are again parsed and strength of each evidence is calculated.
    d. Based on the strength of the evidence all the hypotheses are given a score.
4. Users are now apprised with the solutions in the form of Hypotheses as a list.

Basically, parsing of natural language and scoring of evidence results in evaluating the unstructured text records. Apache UIMA (Unstructured Information Management Architecture) based software components perform those tasks. For each question many search queries are generated, and many different search techniques are used to give the evidence and hypotheses. Different search technologies used are Apache Lucene (term frequency to rank results), Indri (Bayesian network to rank results), and SPARQL (search relationships between terms and documents).

Figure 1. The workflow Watson goes through to answer a question
Source: (http://www.ibm.com/developerworks/library/os-ind-watson/#fig1)

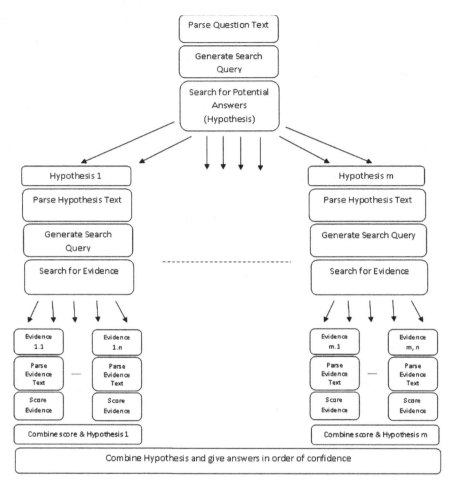

Let's consider a case of an ailment with multiple treatments that can be offered, the Watson service can help patient in deciding the course of treatment to undertake based on the various parameters including chances of success of the treatment, Adverse effects of the treatment opted, planned treatment duration and chances of success to name a few.

IBM Watson provides for an interactive engine to the user for making an optimum choice based on parameters of patient's choice, the same can be ascertained from the figure below.

The Figure 2 gives a snapshot of the possible medications to a certain ailment, detailing each treatment with information on duration of treatment, Adverse affects,

Chances of success, Duration of effectiveness of treatment and cost of the treatment. The patient can now make an informed decision taking into account the various parameters for an effective and suitable treatment.

The Figure 3 provides a visual tool offering interactivity to make suitable choices from the various offered parameters.

Let's consider another example of selection of drug for a certain treatment, Watson would pull out all the possible drugs that can be administered along with details of probability on intestinal absorption, Blood barrier penetration, Non-carcinogenic probability along with other parameters.

The Figure 4 gives a snapshot of the various choices of drugs by Watson with relevant details about the performance of each drug.

The Figure 5 details the choice of the drug using an interactive tool provided by Watson.

TECHNICAL SPECIFICATIONS

Watson is build using Open Source software, mainly. It uses Apache UIMA, Apache Lucene, Indrim and SPARQL. Though built on open software but makes use of its own algorithms.

Figure 2. Choice of treatments suggested by Watson

The list of options to analyze:

Id	Name	⊥ Planned treatment duration (months)	⊥ Adverse effects (1 to 5)	↑ Chance of success (%)	↑ Duration of effectiveness (years)	⊥ Out of pocket expenses ($)
0	BTC	12	5	50	10	8500
1	BIC followed by weekly syntinene	10	3	70	6.5	11000
2	EG followed by syntinene every 2 weeks	7	4	70	15	8750
3	FEG followed by weekly syntinene	7	4	85	14.75	8750
4	EG followed by weekly syntinene	3	1	65	5	8000
5	AG followed by donatel every 3 weeks	10	3	90	6	11000
6	Dose-dense AG followed by donatel	8	5	67	13	7900
7	FEG followed by N	13	2	84	10	10500
8	NBT	13	5	45	10	8500
9	NBT followed by weekly syntinene	11	3	50	6.5	11000
10	ST followed by syntinene every 2 weeks	10	5	60	8	9000
11	GEG followed by weekly syntinene	9	4	60	14.75	8750

Figure 3. Interactive view of treatment selection using Watson

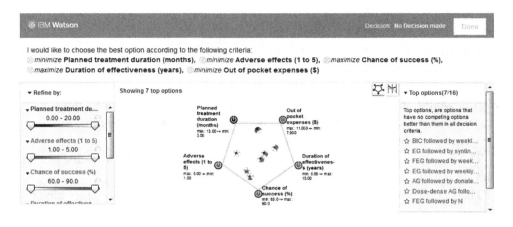

Figure 4. Snapshot of drug choices offered by Watson

The list of options to analyze:

Id	Name	↑ Human Intestinal Absorption (probability)	↑ Blood Brain Barrier Penetration (probability)	⁻ Non-carcinogenic (probability)	↓ Rat acute toxicity (LD50, mol/kg)	↑ Not an hERG inhibitor (probability)
0	Blanfilast	0.991	0.9446	0.875	2.9547	0.7501
1	Prembelol	0.9484	0.8631	0.5199	2.3882	0.8546
2	Glucofilon	0.8589	0.9143	0.9716	3.3039	0.969
3	Thamiphoride	0.9775	0.9382	0.9378	1.2287	0.8735
4	Pseudonarine	0.9645	0.5638	0.7739	2.6024	0.9277
5	Eriladrine	0.9934	0.966	0.9322	2.9371	0.7961
6	Chlorogaline	0.9939	0.7421	0.8374	2.2158	0.8293
7	Eurolone	0.9522	0.9525	0.9116	2.3715	0.7418
8	Tranfilast	0.981	0.9346	0.775	3.2158	0.7501
9	Premvinol	0.9184	0.7631	0.5	3.024	0.8546
10	Glutofilon	0.766	0.8143	0.716	3.4287	0.969
11	Thaminorphoride	0.9375	0.8382	0.9	3.3039	0.735
12	Pseudocitarine	0.6645	0.538	0.5739	2.9882	0.917
13	Xiladrine	0.7934	0.766	0.9322	2.5715	0.7961
14	Ciprogaline	0.8139	0.5421	0.75	2.9547	0.8293
15	Monolone	0.9122	0.9425	0.9	3.0371	0.7418

■ Pre-selected objectives that the service will compare upon clicking Analyze.

↑ An objective that will be maximized.

↓ An objective that will be minimized.

Figure 5. Interactive tool to make selection of drug by Watson

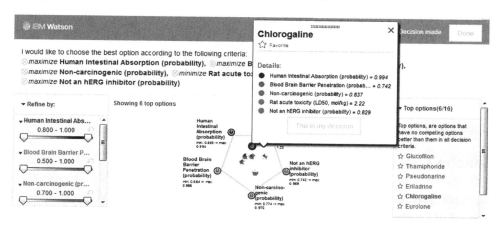

Apache UIMA

To execute the text-process applications like Watson, OASIS UIMA is a useful framework. Apache UIMA is an open source outcome of the OASIS UIMA

It works by creating a link like structure of different applications (called components) in a chain. The results of text processing of one application are passed to the next linked in the chain for further processing.

UIMA-AS is a parallel processing framework, which allows parallel executions of different applications (components). For developing in Java UIMA-AS uses Apache open source framework, ActiveMQ, which uses Java Messaging Services to allow communication between tasks asynchronously.

In Watson, we have already seen after the hypothesis is generated scoring is done.

UIMA-AS made 2880 CPUs to come up with *Jeopardy!* answers within 3 seconds. If so much of resources are not needed then the system can scale down also. As in the case of "physician assistant" application need not to be too fast, which will require lesser amount of resources as compared to Watson.

The unstructured text document if given as input to an annotator (UIMA application) coded in Java or C++, which gives structured information as an output. In order to write these annotators UIMA documentation can be used which hosts a large piece of information having examples also using regular-expressions etc.

In NLP not only extracting of information with regular-expressions is required but large number of algorithms to find, generate tokens, tag, distinguish, and parsing of characters, letters and sentences from the input paragraph to extract its meaning based on the problem is used.

AS UIMA is an open source framework, other developers are encouraged to write their own algorithms and use them. Developers to create the annotators also use many known algorithms; the open source makes it easier to be used by new users. Huge amount of repositories of annotators like OpenNLP (Open Natural Language Processing) and IBM Semantic Search annotators can be downloaded from UIMA website.

To search by a specific name in document repository The IBM Semantic Search annotators is used.

Apache Lucene

We have already seen; to get hypotheses and their supporting evidence a large amount of database is searched. Indexing and searching of the unstructured documents Apache Lucene is used.

It is written in Java with full power of indexing and searching, along with APIs, which allow developers to use it in their own applications. It allows personalization of indexing and scoring as per developer's choice. It also enables to use a high-end query language similar to Google search engine query language

Large documentation repositories: a trivial database and Wikipedia articles for *Jeopardy!* and Lucene indexes medical publications for the health-care application. During questions and answering session UIMA annotators whenever required to search database invoke Lucene. Peer reviewed medical journals like Medline and official guidelines like from Agency for Healthcare Research and Quality makes the examples of database for Lucene.

It stores the structured information generated by UIMA and also indexes the unstructured data based on count of words. Structured data results in a specific format and it enables searching through column fields (metadata). The structured information is stored in Common Analysis Structure (CAS). The Lucene CAS indexer (Lucas) is a standard annotator, which comes along with UIMA. Lucas saves CAS information into Lucene index files.

UIMA and Lucene work together to form the analytics and knowledge engine for Watson.

Mobile Applications

Watson can be used for building health based mobile applications. The cloud API of Watson can be used to develop these mobile applications. The mobile applications make the use very easy by integrating the power of Watson in mobile. User can get the updates on his mobile for all his health related queries. It serves as a full time nurse for the user. We can say it is a digital nurse for the users.

WATSON AND BLUEMIX

Watson services are available on IBM cloud Bluemix. Bluemix is a Platform as a Service (PaaS) from IBM where user can make and deploy applications of various types. With the integration of Watson with Bluemix to develop user based health applications using power of Watson Healthcare has become easier. Watson Application Program Interface (APIs) can be integrated with user's application in a very easy way.

Watson Clinical Trial

According to National Institutes of Health, USA, Clinical trials are the methods to find whether new medical approaches will work fine on people or not. It finds the solutions for diseases and also enables to prevent from diagnosis by answering the questions. It may also analyze a treatment by comparing it with already available treatment.

Watson Clinical Trial is a huge machine learning experience with large amount of data. Here we describe a step-by-step procedure for using clinical trial service of Watson.

Step 1: Register at Watson Clinical Trial (https://apps.admin.ibmcloud.com/account/public/trial/signup?partNumber=CTM_Trial)

This will allow 30-day free trial.

Step 2: Once you login you will get a screen as can be seen in Figure 6.

The diagnosis gives options for five types of Cancer; Colon, Breast, Rectal, Colorectal and Lung Cancer. Choose the required option and fill other details.

Step 3: Once you submit the details as in step 2, the next page opens as shown in Figure 7.

After filling the required details on this screen press on ASK WATSON tab shown in green. Try to enter optional patient data details also, as it would give results that are closer to the concerned patient. Entering the location/zip code also facilitates in the same manner.

Step 4: After entering all the required details. Watson processes the information and gives the results as shown in Figure 8.

Figure 6. Screen Shot for New patient entry

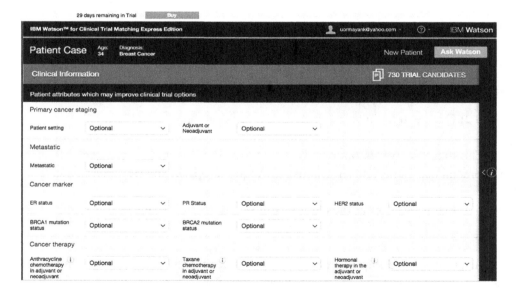

Figure 7. Screen shot for details of patients

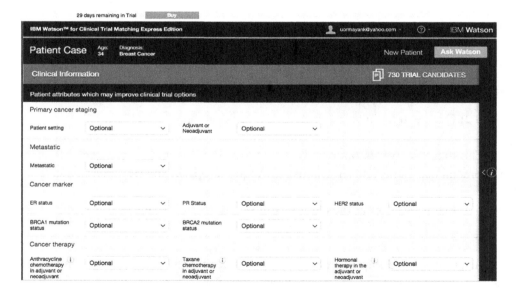

Figure 8. Screen shot of results

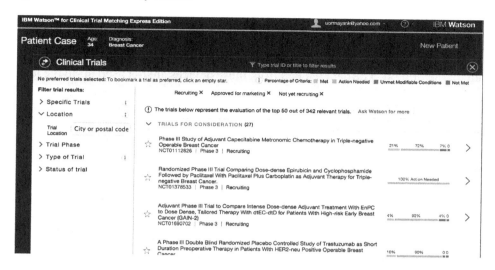

The results (Trials) are divided in two categories Trials for consideration and Ineligible Trials.

Trials for Consideration

This section refers to the trials, which matches with the patient's data and can be considered for further diagnosis. The trials show 4 variations:

- **Met:** In this clinical trial data matches with patient data.
- **Action Needed:** In it Watson requires more input from the patient, to know exactly about suitable clinical trial.
- **Unmet Modifiable Conditions:** In it are the trials which are not met currently with the patient but which might modify at later stage and be useful for the patient.
- **Not Met:** In it are the trials, which are of no use for the patient.

Ineligible Trials

These are the trials for which the patient is not eligible. They have Not Met trials at a higher range.

Step 5: After getting the trials, you can Filter them by clicking on them. You can choose by checking the Action Needed check box and unchecking others to gather all action needed trials. Further on expanding the trials feed additional information to get more results by clicking on Ask Watson tab.

WATSON AND WEARABLE DEVICES

Wearable devices are small devices, which we can wear, and they give us data for different purposes. Mostly wearable devices are used for lifestyle and health related data for egg. Fit bit. The data fetched from these devices are not used up-to the level it can be used because of complex programming and machine learning required in analyzing that data. Watson API gives a way in which this data can be used for much better information and results.

Lack of Information

These wearable's gives lots of data but actual information is still lacking. For example, consider the case of Fit bit which tells you how much calories you have burnt today by walking but it does not cover whether this is good for your health or not depending on your age, and other characteristics and condition.

Bridging the Gap

Watson API helps in bridging these gaps. The data collected from wearable devices is easily integrated with other data and records to give a much clear and better analysis of the data. Currently no such tool is available which allows you to do so with very little programming efforts and without building your own system, Watson is one, which provides you such opportunity.

Watson APIs

Watson has got some few APIs, which are available in Watson Service Catalog. (Sen, 2015). The APIs are:

- Concept Expansion
- Concept Insights
- Language Identification
- Machine Translation
- Message Resonance
- Natural Language Classifier
- Personality Insights
- Question and Answer
- Relationship Extraction
- Speech to Text and Text to Speech
- Tradeoff Analytics

- Visual Recognition
- Visualization Rendering

To make this service more accessible and easier Watson is integrated with Blue-mix the IBM cloud (PaaS). Users can make their applications and integrate Watson services as per their requirements directly in Bluemix. These facilitate them to work on any simple machine connected with Internet and choose the programming language of their choice.

HOW TO USE WATSON API

In this section we consider to use Watson Trade of Analytics APIs. For it we need the following:

- A Bluemix account
- The Cloud Foundry CLI tool
- Basic understanding of JavaScript
- Basic understanding of Node.js

Step-by-Step method to deploy the application using CLI tool is explained below:

1. Get the Tradeoff Analytics Node.js application from GitHub (https://github.com/watson-developer-cloud/tradeoff-analytics-nodejs) in one of these ways:
   ○ Download the .zip file and unpack it to a directory called Try
   ○ If you are using Git, clone the repo to the Try directory
2. Navigate to the Try directory, and then edit the manifest.yml file.
3. Log in to IBM Bluemix by entering the following command from the Try directory where you downloaded the source code:

```
cf login -a https://api.ng.bluemix.net.
```

4. Provide your login credentials, and if you have more than one workspace, select a workspace.
5. Push the code up to IBM Bluemix by entering the following command:

```
cf push Try -no-start
```

6. Create an instance of the Tradeoff Analytics service by entering the following command:cf create-service tradeoff_analytics standard tradeoff_analytics_node.js.

7. Bind the service instance to the Try application instance by entering the following command:

```
cf bind-service Try.tradeoff_analytics_nodejs
```

8. Restage the application by entering the following command:

```
cf restage Try
```

9. Log in to your Bluemix account.
10. Open the user interface for your Try application by using one of these methods:
    ○ Copy the route or URL that displays under the application name.
    ○ Click the *open website* button, under your Try application, which is next to the running text.

FUTURE OF NATURAL LANGUAGE PROCESSING IN HEALTHCARE

Natural language processing in health-care is much more that doubts and solutions. In 2008, the Nature journal published an issue indicating on how big data can be used for medical purposes. The medical science is moving towards data mining for conclusions rather than theoretical and hypothetical views. Genomic data is used big data mining in Nature but natural language text data is can also be used, ant it opens a research front using text data.

We can take the digital records of doctor's notes as input for big data mining to give treatment options, symptom based diagnosis, reductions in medical errors etc. Mayo Clinic has already tied up with IBM to give its records to be used and searched by using Watson and integrate it with UIMA annotators.

Not only the doctor's data but also feedback from patients, their blogs, and emails can also be used for data mining to help in medical analysis. Communities like Patients LikeMe and Association of Cancer Online Resources have large amount of this type of data. The reports of patients telling about adverse effects of medicines not covered by FDA and also sometimes the solutions given are patients can be mined for better treatments. Natural language tools, can take medical Science to new heights.

By Open-Source and Cloud based hardware, Watson shows what can be done. The open source and easy deployable efforts by R&D team of Watson has given an opportunity to the developer community to write innovative applications to take advantage of these capabilities!

FUTURE RESEARCH DIRECTIONS

IBM Watson can be integrated with any medical issues, the user can built his own IoT applications for any illness he wishes to, as there are no restrictions from Watson. Recently IBM tied with Apple and Apple watch intenerated with Watson to predict the health status in depending on sleeping habit.

CONCLUSION

The average life span in 2014 is reported to be 64 years, in 1869 it was 26 years, in 1800 it was 23 years, with the advent of antibiotics the life span increased 3 times in 150 years and with the advent of IT and cloud computing with the help of Watson we can expect life span of 90 years within short span of time. Think is it possible for a doctor to record details of $5 * 10^{30}$ bacteria moving in the atmosphere. But with Watson it is possible.

Watson's way of reasoning is to generate hypotheses (that is, candidate answers) from a large body of documents, as opposed to from pre-conceived theories as humans typically do. In fact, a major trend in scientific research is to "mine" discoveries from data. While Watson is trying to emulate human intelligence, humans seem to think more like Watson too!

REFERENCES

Best, J. (2011). IBM Watson the Inside Story. *Tech Republic*. Retrieved January 21, 2016, from http://www.techrepublic.com/article/ibm-watson-the-inside-story-of-how-the-jeopardy-winning-supercomputer-was-born-and-what-it-wants-to-do-next/

Debroha, D. (2015). IBM Watson Health Announces New Partnership. *IBM PR Newswire*. Retrieved January 20, 2016, from http://www.prnewswire.com/news/ibm+watson+health

Feldman, S., & Handover, J. (2012). Unlocking the Power of Unstructured Data. *IDC Health Insights*. Retrieved January 21, 2016, from http://www01.ibm.com/software/ebusiness/jstart /downloads/unlockingUnstructuredData.pdf

Macmillan, R., & Dowskin, E. (2015). IBM Crafts a Role for Artificial Intelligence. *Wall Street Journal*. Retrieved January 20, 2016, from http://www.wsj.com/articles/ibm-craftsaroleforartificialintelligenceinmedicine1439265840

National Institutes of Health. (n.d.). *Mediline Plus*. Retrieved February 23, 2016, from www.nlm.nih.gov/medlineplus/clinicaltrials.html

Sen, R. (2015). Building smarter wearable's for health-care. *IBM Developer Works*. Retrieved January 15, 2016, from http://www.ibm.com/developerworks/library/cc-smarter-wearables-healthcare-concepts/index.html

KEY TERMS AND DEFINITIONS

Bluemix: A PaaS by IBM.

Cloud: It is a model that provides access/compute/storage to users any time any place and on any device connected by Internet.

IoT: A device connected and controlled through Internet irrespective of the location.

Mobile Applications: Applications, which are made for, and run on mobile devices are called mobile applications.

Chapter 8
Data Protection and Security Issues in Social Media

Chintan M. Bhatt
Charotar University of Science and Technology, India

ABSTRACT

Cloud Computing changes the way Information Technology (IT) is expended and oversaw, promising enhanced cost efficiencies, quickened advancement, quicker time-to-market, and the capacity to scale applications of interest (Leighton, 2009). Users have started to explore new ways to interact with each other with the omnipresent nature of Social Networks and Cloud Computing. Facebook, YouTube, Orkut, Twitter, Flickr, Google+, Four Square, Pinterest, and the likes have distorted the way the Internet (Social Cloud) is being used. However, there is an absence of comprehension of protection and security issues of online networking. The protection and security of online networking should be explored, concentrated on and portrayed from different viewpoints (PCs, social, mental and so on). It is basic to distinguish security dangers and shield protection through constant and adaptable frameworks. Subsequent to there is no intelligent limits of the social networking, it is vital to consider the issue from a worldwide viewpoint as well.

DOI: 10.4018/978-1-5225-1002-4.ch008

INTRODUCTION

Social Networking implies the technique for relationship among people in which they make, offer, and/or trade data and thoughts in virtual groups and systems. Over each industry, numerous organizations are thinking that it's vital to have a vicinity on one or more online networking channels, for example, Facebook, XING, LinkedIn, foursquare, MySpace, YouTube, Wikipedia and Twitter. Online networking is a social association where the clients are aloof buyers, as well as have an immediate correspondence with the organization.

Social Networks contain an abundance of data. These include:

- Date of Birth
- Email address
- Home address
- Family ties
- Pictures

Social Media is defined as "a group of Internet-based applications that build on the ideological and technological foundations of Web 2.0 and that allow the creation and exchange of user-generated content". The potential uses of social media correspond to a wide scope of lawful issues. The main purpose of chapter *is to discuss various issues regarding security and protection of data in social networking and possible solutions.*

BACKGROUND

Disregarding the few points of interest that Cloud Computing carries alongside it, there are a few concerns and issues which should be fathomed before omnipresent appropriation of this processing worldwide happens. To begin with, in distributed computing, the client might not have the sort of control over his/her information or the execution of his/her applications that he/she might require, or the capacity to review or change the procedures and approaches under which he/she should work. Diverse parts of an application may be in a better place in the cloud that can adversely affect the execution of the application. Consenting to regulations might be troublesome, particularly when discussing cross-out skirt issues – it ought to likewise be noticed that the regulations still should be created to consider all parts of distributed computing. It is entirely common that checking and upkeep is not as straightforward an undertaking when contrasted with what it is really going after sitting in the Intranet. Second, the cloud clients might hazard having so as to lose information they bolted into restrictive configurations and might lose control over their information since the apparatuses for observing who is utilizing them or who can see them are not generally gave to the clients. Information misfortune is, accordingly, a possibly genuine danger in some particular arrangements. Third, it may not be anything but difficult to tailor administration level assertions (SLAs) to the particular needs of a business. Pay for downtime might be insufficient and SLAs are unrealistic to cover the corresponding harms. It is sensible to adjust the expense of ensuring inward uptime against the benefits of selecting the cloud. From the point of view of the associations, having next to zero capital venture might really have charge burdens. From the point of view of the associations, having next to zero capital venture might really have charge drawbacks. At long last, the measures are youthful and looking for taking care of the quickly changing and developing advanced of distributed computing. Thusly, one can't simply move applications to the cloud and anticipate that they will run effectively. At long last, there are idleness and execution issues following the Internet associations and the system connections might add to inertness or might put limitations on the accessible data transfer capacity.

Issue: Old Security Models vs. New Enterprise IT Models

IT security has endured with a static, area based and firm design, however venture IT has continually turned out to be more dynamic, portable, open, outward-confronting and collective. Accordingly, when clients go "versatile", they are rebuffed by the framework since they can no more get to the same applications. Static security is less receptive to change; more perplexing and vulnerable to the presentation of human mistake. Organizations need to modify their security framework and present a character driven design which offers changing, adaptable, portable, strategy based security. This research work is documented in the work of Andreas M. Antonopoulos (2011).

DATA PROTECTION AND SECURITY IN SOCIAL MEDIA

Data Protection Basics

The Data Protection Act 1998 (United Kingdom Act of Parliament, March 2000) sets up a structure of rights and obligations which are intended to ensure individual information. It adjusts the honest to goodness needs of associations to gather and utilize individual information for business and different purposes against the privilege of people to regard for the protection of their own points of interest. This work is documented in Data Protection Principles, ico. The Data Protection Act 1998

(DPA) depends on eight standards of "good data taking care of" which information controllers are required to conform to. In practice, it means that you must:

- Have a true blue reason for gathering and utilizing the individual information.
- Not utilize the information in ways that have unjustified unfavorable consequences for the people concerned.
- Be straightforward about how you expect to utilize the information, and give people suitable security sees when gathering their own information.
- Handle individuals' close to home information just in ways they would sensibly anticipate.
- Ensure you don't do anything unlawful with the information.

Fair Processing of Data

Processing personal data must satisfy the pertinent conditions for processing.

Processing broadly means collecting, using, disclosing, retaining or disposing of personal data, and if any aspect of processing is unfair, there will be a breach of the first data protection principle – even if you can show that you have met one or more of the conditions for processing.
Fairness generally requires you to be transparent – clear and open to individuals about how their information will be used.

Surveying whether data is being handled reasonably depends halfway on how it is gotten. The Data Protection Act says that data ought to be dealt with as being gotten reasonably in the event that it is given by a man who is lawfully approved or required, to give it.

Case: Personal information will be acquired reasonably by the assessment powers in the event that it is gotten from a business who is under a legitimate obligation to give points of interest of a representative's pay, regardless of whether the worker agrees to, or knows about, this.

Nonetheless, to evaluate regardless of whether individual information is handled decently, you should consider all the more by and large how it influences the hobbies of the general population concerned – as a gathering and separately. On the off chance that the data has been getting and utilized reasonably as a part of connecting to a large portion of the general population, it identifies with yet unjustifiably in connection to one individual, there will be a break of the main information security guidelines.

Personal information might here and there be utilized as a part of a way that causes some disservice to (adversely influences) a person without this essentially being unjustifiable.

Case: Where personal data is collected to charge tax liability or to compel a fine for breaking the speed limit, the data is being utilized as a part of a way that might make disadvantage the people concerned, yet the correct utilization of individual information for these reasons won't be out of line.

A few associations offer personal information with different associations. For instance, foundations working in the same field might wish to utilize or share supporters' data to permit proportional mailings. A few organizations, even exchange personal information, offering or leasing the data. The people concerned should in any case be dealt with reasonably. They ought to be informed that their data might be shared, so they can pick regardless of whether to go into an association with the association sharing it.

Why and how personal information is gathered and utilized will be applied as a part of evaluating decency.

Reasonableness requires to:

- Be transparent about identity.
- Advise individuals how to utilize any personal information which is gathered about them (unless this is self-evident).
- Normally handle their own information just in ways they would sensibly anticipate.
- Most importantly, not utilize their data in ways that ridiculously negatively affect them.

Privacy Notices

The Data Protection Act does not define reasonable preparing. In any case, it says that, unless a significant exclusion applies, individual information will be handled genuinely just if certain data is given to the individual or people concerned. It is clear that the law gives associations some circumspection by the way they give reasonable preparing data – extending from effectively conveying it to making it promptly accessible.

In general terms, a privacy notice ought to state:

- Your personality and on the off chance that you are not situated in the INDIA, the character of your designated INDIA agent

- The reason or purposes for which you mean to prepare the data
- Any additional data you have to give people in the circumstances to empower you to handle the data decently.

The remainder of these necessities is dubious. Be that as it may, on the grounds that the Data Protection Act covers a wide range of preparing, it is difficult to be prescriptive. At the point when choosing whether you ought to give some other data in light of a legitimate concern for reasonableness, you need to consider the way of the individual information and what the people concerned are liable to anticipate. For instance, on the off chance that you mean to unveil data to another association, reasonableness requires that you tell the people concerned unless they are prone to expect such divergences. It is additionally great practice to tell individuals how they can get to the data you hold about them, as this might help them spot mistakes or exclusions in their records.

At the point when choosing how to draft and impart a security notice, endeavor to place yourself in the position of the all inclusive community you are social event information about.

Ask yourself:

- Do they definitely know who is gathering the data and what it will be utilized for?
- Is there anything they would discover tricky, deluding, startling or questionable?
- Are the results of giving the information, or not giving it, clear to them?

Case: At the point when an individual goes into a cellular telephone contract, they know the cell telephone organization will keep their name and address subtle elements for charging purposes. This does not should be spelt out. Be that as it may, if the organization needs to utilize the data for another reason, maybe to empower a sister organization to make occasion offers, then this would not be evident to the individual client and ought to be disclosed to them.

Lawful

Lawful refers to the *statute and to common law, whether criminal or civil*. However, processing may be unlawful if it results in:

- A rupture of an obligation of certainty. Such an obligation might be expressed, or it might be suggested by the substance of the data or in light of the fact that it was gathered in circumstances where secrecy is normal.

- Your association surpassing its legitimate powers or practicing those forces shamefully.
- An encroachment of copyright
- A rupture of an enforceable contract ascension
- A rupture of industry-particular enactment or regulations
- A violation of the Human Rights Act 1998. The Act actualizes the European Convention on Human Rights which, in addition to other things, gives people the privilege to regard for private and family life, home and correspondence.

Because of the way that the data posted on the interpersonal organizations' sites turn out to be for the most part open to general society, we need to pay additional consideration to the data that we unveil about us, which basically, by getting to be known not expansive number of individuals can prompt the "creation of a risk to privacy or even to the physical safety of a person".

A website which permits posting individual information must guarantee the security of the data and not to be utilized for different purposes. A large portion of these sites permits the setting of the data which is being posted as open or private data, by utilizing the control choice "security settings". In the event that a percentage of the sites are mechanized set at a private level, for others you need to pick this alternative in an express way.

It is prescribed to those utilizing the social network sites:

- To abstain from posting of individual data such as the location or telephone number
- To abstain from utilizing certain passwords which can be effortlessly recognized, even by shut persons
- To utilize a unique email address, not the same as the individual or expert one.

Each organization has diverse online networking objectives. Intel Corporation, for instance, traces three key rules of engagement in online networking rules for its representatives:

1. Disclose: Presence in social media must be crystal clear.
2. Protect: take an additional concern to protect both Intel and yourself.
3. Use Common Sense: keep in mind that professional, simple, and suitable communication is best.

Mrs. Georgeta Basarabescu - president of the NATIONAL SUPERVISORY AUTHOR-ITY - worries the way that the informal organizations suppliers ought to gather and process touchy information (concerning the racial or ethnic starting point, political, religious, philosophical convictions, exchange union fidelity, individual information in regards to the condition of wellbeing or sexual coexistence) just with the communicated and unequivocal assent of the information subject, as per the perspective of Article 29 Working Party as its would see it no. 5/2009.

This worldwide record expresses that the informal organization suppliers ought to set up the maintenance time of idle clients' information, and the records surrendered must be erased.

DATA SECURITY: TOP THREATS TO DATA PROTECTION

The Data Protection Act says that:

Appropriate technical and organizational measures shall be taken against unauthorized or unlawful processing of personal data and against accidental loss or destruction of, or damage to, personal data.

According to 7th Data Protection Principle, anyone must have suitable security to thwart the personal data. In particular, anyone will need to:

- Plan and deal with security to fit the method for the individual data he/she hold and the wickedness that may happen due to a security break.
- Be clear about who in affiliation is accountable for ensuring information/data security.
- Ensure he/she has the privilege physical and specialized security.
- Be arranged to respond to any break of security rapidly and adequately.

Data Security strategy is essential to:

1. Ensure passwords are not shared
2. Ensure access to hostile destinations is averted on work frameworks
3. Make clear practices which are despicable
4. Delineate the general population and private areas for the reasons of the work framework and disperse desires of protection
5. Ensure that the results of rupture are caught on

Delineations of the naughtiness brought on by the hardship or abuse of individual data (Sometimes associated with character extortion) include:

- Fake charge card exchanges
- Witnesses in danger of physical damage or intimidation
- Offenders at danger from vigilantes
- Exposure of the locations of administration staff, police and jail officers and ladies at danger of abusive behavior at home
- Fake applications for assessment credits
- Mortgage misrepresentation.

Comprehend that the essentials of the Data Protection Act go past the way information is secured or transmitted. The seventh data confirmation standard relates to the security of every piece of your treatment of individual data. So the endeavors to build up wellbeing you put set up should hope to ensure that:

- Just affirmed people can get the chance to, conform or demolish singular data
- Those people simply act within the degree of their energy
- On the remote possibility that the individual data is accidentally lost, changed or crushed, it can be recovered to keep any damage or inconvenience to the general population concerned.

Be that as it may, when security can't adjust to change, it turns into a perpetual killjoy, backing off change and step by step making the business less and less aggressive. Organizations that can resolve this "unimaginable decision" can turn security from an obstruction to an empowering influence of progress. An adaptable and element security foundation permits security officers to say "YES" to versatility, to tablets, to blend, to joint effort and to fast application arrangement, while notwithstanding diminishing danger.

Movements in Information Technology (IT) have raised stresses over the perils of data associated with delicate IT security, including vulnerability to contaminations, malware, attacks and deal of framework systems and organizations. To guarantee that individual protection remains painstakingly ensured, nearby and state training offices ought to actualize best in class data security hones. Staying in front of the constantly advancing danger of an information break requires persistence with respect to the training group in comprehension and envisioning the dangers. Dangers are separated into two classifications: specialized and non-specialized. When in doubt, an association can extraordinarily diminish its weakness to the security dangers by actualizing an extensive protection and information security arrangement.

Security Threats for Personal / Profile Information

Email addresses from databases can be utilized for spam crusaders. *TrendLabs* scientists have reported costs of individual data running from US$50 per stolen financial balance accreditations to about US$8 per million email addresses. This last figure is liable to be much higher in the event that it includes crisp locations. Date of Birth information is utilized by various organizations to affirm individuals' personalities via phone. Crooks have devices to robotize "date of conception" inquiries in interpersonal interaction destinations.

Another element that fuels this huge information spillage potential is a client's open profile. At the point when clients set their data to be available without signing into the long range informal communication site, that data can be recorded in web indexes or some other chronicle. There are informal communication web search tools that can look all accessible information about any name in a specific district. This makes the lives of stalkers, fraudsters, or some other aggressor much less demanding. Not just do a Google and different crawlers assemble openly accessible data, however, there are likewise meta-web indexes like pipl.com particularly intended to pursuit long range interpersonal communication locales and different sources to accumulate a wide range of data.

It is simple for miscreants to create a large network of contacts by using any number of techniques such as:

- Making a fake VIP profile and allowing individuals to add them to their contact records
- Making a duplicate of someone's profile and re-respecting the greater part of their companions
- Making a profile, adding themselves to a medium-sized gathering and respecting various individuals from the gathering (colleges, schools, social orders and so forth.). At that point joining a second gathering and starting once more.
- Making a female profile and distributed a beautiful picture of "herself". Numerous individuals use long range interpersonal communication locales to meet their accomplices online and countless have particular devices to help with this.

There are various systems that permit an aggressor to break the circle of trust and get into individual contact records. A great deal of interpersonal organization clients doesn't understand that their contact records truly are a circle of trust and by including some person they don't know—VIPs included—they are opening their information to untrusted.

A few locals don't have security controls set up, or the ones they don't ensure all client information. Regardless of the possibility that they do have far reaching protection controls, the client is regularly not committed to choosing who can get to his/her information and is frequently discouraged from utilizing the accessible controls since they show up excessively mind boggling or tedious. Numerous clients basically don't try to design these controls, be it for lethargy or absence of information. This implies whether by the website's outline or the client's absence of interest, individual information is unnecessarily presented to outsiders, internet searchers, and the more extensive online world.

With a large network, following threats can be possible:

One option is advertising. By composing/remarking on individuals' profiles or sending private mail, the assailant can appropriate connections promoting sites and items. On the off chance that this procedure is done quietly, it can work generally well, albeit ordinarily this will be an excess of exertion for any aggressor. Contacts will rapidly see that the posts are secret publicizing and will erase/obstruct the aggressor inside and out.

The same can be refined by private Web Messaging, which every social webpage permits, however it is also ineffectual for the same reasons expressed previously. These sorts of long range informal communication spam runs are more often than not of an exceptionally restricted length of time and originate from pay-per-snap or pay-per-activity associate based web promoting plans.

The second choice is the social event of contact data, for instance, email addresses or phone numbers. Those social destinations that show your companions' contact data can be used to accumulate working email databases alongside telephone numbers (or other information that can serve to better target future spam, and phishing effort). There are individuals assembling huge contact databases, which are later sold to spammers, con artists, and Visa fraudsters. The estimation of such a database is measured on the nature of the information. More prepared email databases have been spammed over and over so the locations may have been tossed. The more vital email databases consolidate new working messages, (for example, the ones you can discover on long range informal communication destinations). This kind of data is useful for directing effort and can be sold through the underground economy.

The third option is for phishing and/or malware fixing. Envision this situation—the assailant makes a phishing page indistinguishable to Facebook's login page. At that point they change their status line to "check this entertaining video I discovered yesterday" and a connection to the fake page. At the point when individuals tap the connection, they are given a fake Facebook login page, which they use to "sign in" once more, maybe imagining that some way or another their session had timed out. As of right now, the assailant has the casualty's username and secret word, however the assault does not end there. In the wake of "signing in," the fake page shows an entertaining video that adventures program helplessness and introduces a Trojan out of sight. This is not a theoretical situation, but rather an abnormal state depiction of the exercises of the malware known as "KOOBFACE" that have been victorious spreading on various informal communities.

This is the authentic danger of social and group based destinations—clients trust their contacts to not send horrible associations, to not to endeavor to pollute their PCs and take extraordinary thought of their own data. Once the trust is broken any of those circumstances can happen whenever.

The genuine artfulness originates from masking those terrible connections as though they were great. A typical client will most likely have no issue tapping on a youtube.com join originating from an online contact, however may be more cautious with a badsite.org join. Enter URL shorteners. These online redirec¬tion benefits intentionally conceal a URL so as to make it shorter. Conceal vindictive URLs don't look dangerous before tapping on them. After that snap, however, it is frequently past the point of no return. These shortening administrations are so broadly utilized that individuals don't reconsider before clicking one of them, even without recognizing what prowls behind.

Social networking sites keep adding to their security controls and refining their current ones in any case, as in any improvement venture, they additionally keep on developing on their stages and add energizing new components. These new alternatives need to stay aware of the security components or they too will experience the ill effects of security shortcomings.

Technical Data Security Threats to Information Systems

Nonexistent Security Architecture

A few associations have not set up security set up set up, helpless against misuse and the loss of eventually identifiable information (PII). From time to time, in view of a nonattendance of benefits or qualified IT staff, affiliations' frameworks are connected with the web particularly, or are related using out-of-the-container framework mechanical assemblies with default setups joined, with no additional layer of protection. It is basic to note that having a firewall alone is not sufficient to ensure the security of a framework. Deficient framework protection results in extended shortcoming of the data, hardware, and programming, including frailty to vindictive programming (malware), diseases, and hacking. If the framework contains unstable information or PII, for instance, understudies' institutionalized investment fund numbers, it is critical that even in an incredibly obliged resource environment, irrelevant customer, framework and edge security protection segments, (for instance, threatening to contamination) are executed, including guaranteeing that against disease writing computer programs is properly planned. Generous security outline is major and gives a manual for executing indispensable information insurance measures.

Mitigation: In the event that an affiliation does not have the suitable workforce to layout security designing, it is proposed that a outsider be obtained to guide with the IT bun.

Un-Patched Client Side Software and Applications

PCs run a collection of programming applications, including more settled versions of that may now and again contain vulnerabilities that can be manhandled by noxious performing craftsmen. Staying mindful of programming upgrades and overhauls, despite applying maker recommended patches, minimizes a substantial number of the vulnerabilities.

Mitigation: To diminish the capacity of malicious actors to trade off or wreck an association's security framework, execute a strong patch administration program that recognizes defenseless programming applications and routinely redesigns the product security to guarantee constant security from well-known threats.

"Phishing" and Targeted Attacks ("Spear Phishing")

One way pernicious people or programmers target individuals and relationship to access individual data is through messages containing malevolent code—this is implied as phishing. Once tainted messages are opened, the customer's machine can be traded.

Mitigation: To decrease defenselessness to phishing and other email security tricks, associations ought to introduce proficient endeavor level email security programming. It is suggested that this software check both approaching and active messages to guarantee that spam messages are not being transmitted if a framework gets to be traded off. What's more, associations ought to give consistent web security training to staff to guarantee client mindfulness about email tricks.

Internet Web Sites

Malicious code can be traded to a PC through skimming WebPages that have not experienced security overhauls. Thus, essentially skimming the web and going to be exchanged off or unsecured locals could achieve dangerous writing computer programs being downloaded to an affiliation's PCs and the framework.

Mitigation: To keep risks from bartered destinations, use firewalls and antivirus programming to perceive and piece perhaps unsafe pages.

Poor Configuration Management

Any PC connected with the framework, whether at work or at home, that does not take after setup organization system, is powerless against an attack. Slight data security protection measures that don't restrain which machines can take up with the affiliation's framework make it defenseless against this sort of danger.

Mitigation: Establish a setup administration procedure for interfacing any hardware to the framework. The plan should decide security frameworks and procedure for various sorts of gear, including PCs, printers, and frameworks organization contraptions. It is additionally prescribed to actualize a Network Access Control answer for upholding setup approach prerequisites (e.g., via naturally anticipating system access to the gadgets that don't conform to the system security arrangements).

Mobile Devices

Use of PDAs, for instance, versatile workstations or handheld contraptions, including propelled cellular telephones, are impacting; regardless, the ability to secure them is waiting behind. The situation is convoluted by the way that these devices are every now and again used to direct work outside the affiliation's standard framework security limits. Data breaks can happen in different ways: devices can be lost, stolen, or their security can be exchanged off by malignant code assaulting the working structure and applications.

Mitigation: To advance information security in the event that a gadget is lost or stolen, scramble information on every single cell phone putting away touchy data (i.e., information that conveys the danger for harm1 from an unapproved). Until more data encryption, customer acceptance, and threatening to malware plans get the chance to be open for PDAs, the best protection framework is to execute a strict mobile phone use approach and screen the framework for malevolent activity.

Cloud Computing

Designating the main part of data protection service to a third party shifts enterprise security architecture. In cloud computing, for instance, a lot of client information is put away in shared assets, which raise an assortment of information encryption and accessibility issues. Further, the cloud supplier confronts the same information security obligations and difficulties as the association that possess the information, including fixing and dealing with their applications against vindictive code.

Mitigation: Conduct an appraisal to look at the advantages of embracing distributed computing, including cost investment funds and expanded effectiveness, against related security dangers. It is basic to guarantee that arrangements offered by the cloud supplier viably conform to the association's data framework security prerequisites, including operational and hazard administration strategies. As cloud arrangements and security necessities keep on advancing, occasionally audit the money saving advantage appraisal.

Removable Media

The use of removable media (e.g., streak drives, CDs, and outside hard drives) confronts a basic security hazard. These sorts of media give a pathway to malware to move between frameworks or hosts. Taking after the proper security measure (while using removable media devices) is critical to decrease the threat of polluting affiliation's machines or the entire framework.

Mitigation: To minimize the security dangers, apply straightforward safeguard steps. These incorporate debilitating the "auto run" highlight of the working framework on the association's machines and preparing clients to examine removable media for infections before opening the records.

Here, damage alludes to any unfriendly impacts that would be experienced by a person whose PII was the subject of lost classification, and in addition any unfavorable impacts experienced by the association that keeps up the PII (NIST, Guide to Protecting the Confidentiality of Personally Identifiable Information (PII). Mischief to an individual incorporates any negative or undesirable impacts (i.e., that might be socially, physically, or fiscally harming).

Botnets

Botnets are frameworks of exchanged off PCs used by software engineers for harmful purposes, by and large criminal in nature. It is the affiliation's commitment to prompt accomplices around a potential exchange off of all data harping on the framework (paying little mind to whether the information themselves were the objective) in the wake of tainting the association's system. Tidy up endeavors coming about because of botnet infestation might be expensive and harming to an association's notoriety. Exploits can take many forms such as *Distributed Denial of Service (DDoS) Attacks, Spyware and Malware, Identity Theft, Adware, Email Spam* etc. Figure 1 shows a typical botnet.

Mitigation: Since there are numerous ways PCs can get to be traded off, having a solid security architecture is basic to protecting against a vindictive botnet assault. Actualize an all encompassing way to deal with information security and use precaution measures to guarantee that the system is secure. Procedures for botnet recognition include breaking down examples of information sent over the system,

Figure 1. A typical botnet with zombies

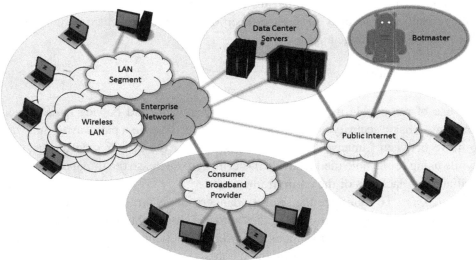

and checking PC assets use and outside associations. The common techniques are *Flow data monitoring, Anomaly detection, DNS log analysis, Honeypots* etc.

Zero-Day Attacks

A zero-day assault is a danger went for abusing programming application weakness before the application trader gets the opportunity to be aware of it and before the frailty ends up being for the most part known not web security bunch. These attacks are among the hardest to mitigate and leave PCs and frameworks to an incredible degree frail.

Mitigation: Unless an affiliation has admitted to IT inspectors who are exceedingly experienced in the specific powerlessness assessment, an as frequently as could be allowed endorsed approach to manage control is to sit tight for the shipper to release a patch that fixes the shortcoming. The affiliation should stay up and coming with the latest programming settles and pass on the fix when it is appropriated by the specialist. This work is documented in Data Security: Top Threats to Data Protection, 2011.

NonTechnical Cyber Security Threats to Information Systems

Insider

An insider is described as some person with real access to the framework. Since information got to by insiders can be easily stolen, imitated, deleted or changed, insider risks can be indisputably the most hurting, paying little regard to whether they happen in view of customer rudeness or threatening tries.

Mitigation: To ease this kind of threat, set up and actualize an inside and out portrayed advantage rights organization structure, keeping customers' passage to certain information and allowing them to simply perform specific limits. Review Programs are important in executing access controls and watching suspicious development.

Poor Passwords

Executing a methodology on strong customer passwords is essential to data security. It is especially basic for customers with access to the most tricky information. Current mystery key part tasks can without quite a bit of a stretch break slight passwords, for instance, those containing essential words or word groups found in a lexicon. Therefore, the customer picked passwords are all around thought to be weaker than heedlessly made passwords. The Client made passwords routinely take after an expected illustration or relationship to something in the customer's life (city, family, or pet names for occurrence) and are thusly all the more helpless against mystery word part extends. While subjectively delivered passwords may be harder to remember that, they are by and large more secure.

Mitigation: Use a specialist mystery word making program as an endeavor level course of action. A collection of uncommonly assessed activities are open accessible. Despite executing systems for delivering strong passwords, train customers on the most capable technique to keep up the security of their passwords, which joins not keeping created passwords in the district of the PC. For enhanced security, consider realizing more impelled acceptance capacities.

Physical Security

Physical security is fundamental to evade unapproved access to fragile data and what's more guaranteeing an affiliation's personnel and resources. A convincing physical security system is a vital part of a broad security program. Physical wellbeing measures join securing access to dedicated PCs, server rooms, switches, printers, and any ranges that methodology or store sensitive data.

Mitigation: Build up and maintain a physical security structure. Strong physical security consolidates access control methodologies and procedures; physical limits (e.g., divider, gateways, locks, safes, etc.); perception and alert structures; and security break cautioning, response, and system recovery frameworks.

Insufficient Backup and Recovery

Nonappearance of an overwhelming data fortification and recovery course of action drives an affiliation's data in threat. Data and system recovery limits allow a relationship to decrease the risk of damage associated with a data crack. It is critical to direct routine fortifications of essential data and store support media in an ensured and secure way.

Mitigation: Build up a various leveled system and demonstrate procedures for data fortification, stockpiling, and recuperation. Various pushed data and structural support and recovery mechanical assemblies are openly accessible.

Improper Destruction

Paper files, for instance, reports and inventories, may contain unstable data. Unless these reports are destroyed fittingly (for case, by pulverizing or blazing), they may be safeguarded and mishandled. Discarded electronic devices, for instance, PCs or reduced drives, that has been used as a piece of taking care of and securing sensitive data, stays feeble unless the data are destroyed properly.

Mitigation: Build up a strategy for securing or crushing no more required IT resources and media that might contain delicate information. A few gauges associations offer rules that diagram best practices for guaranteeing information are disposed of legitimately (including proposals distributed PTAC-IB, by the National Institute of Standards and Technology (NIST) titled NIST SP 800-88) "Rules for Media Sanitization."

Social Media

Using affiliation's devices and framework advantages for getting to internet organizing destinations speaks to a high data security hazard. Long range interpersonal correspondence destinations are routinely engaged by malware, get an abnormal state of spam, and are as regular as could reasonably be expected used to get information for wholes.

Mitigation: Present and sustain a methodology denying access to some web organizing destinations while using an affiliation's benefits and equipment. Train customers about the security perils made by passing by these destinations. Affiliations that allow access to internet organizing destinations should send a strong against disease and spam isolating.

Social Engineering

Breaking into a framework does not require specific aptitudes. Access to tricky information can be grabbed by controlling true blue customers resulting to securing their trust. Caution should be urged when bestowing any record or framework information. This incorporates guaranteeing the requester is comprehended by the customer and has a true clarification behind this information. Socially composed strikes are the strategies for a couple of software engineers to get passwords, access codes, IP areas, switch or server names, and other information that can be abused to break into a framework.

Mitigation: Train customers to grow their care about social planning risks and teach them on the most ideal approach to refuse being controlled. Case in point, customers should be advised to use ready when someone gets some information about their record information or specific information about the framework, especially if this individual cases to be a framework official. This work is documented in Data Security: Top Threats to Data Protection, 2011.

Self-XSS, Clickjecking in Facebook

Facebook is an article for tricks because of a substantial number of clients. Keep in mind "facebook profits from its sponsors, not clients". Facebook offers your data past your gathering of companions. The most recent sample is facebook's facial acknowledgment innovation.

Facebook tricks incorporate cross-site scripting, clickjecking, study tricks, fraud and so on. One of the con artist's most loved techniques for assault on minute is cross-site scripting or "Self-XSS". Such assaults can run covered up and can do malware establishment (with JavaScript) without client's information. Illustration is Facebook Dislike catch which takes client to a site page that tries to deceive him/her into cutting and sticking a malevolent JavaScript code into program's location bar.

Other assault is clickjecking or likejecking. It is otherwise called "UI readdressing". This pernicious strategy traps web clients into uncovering classified data or takes control of their PC when they tap on apparently harmless website pages. It takes the type of implanted code or script that can execute without the client's information. Illustration is Baby Born Amazing impacts.

Recommendations to Improve Social Media Security

Does person to person communication break the dividers of your system security? Today the need to safeguard against information spillage and malware develops more dire.

Possibly your organization as of now does "social business" perceiving that online journals, Twitter, and YouTube are crucial to its deals and brand.

The Risks

At the point when workers tweet, blog, and post, who do they offer data to? A significant part of the information they put on social destinations is posted freely. Other information opens up to the world virtually. The data is constantly held by the site support, for quite a long time. It might likewise be followed by government organizations. Information leaks, and insider facts are given away.

What do workers get from online networking? Infrequently it's more than a relationship based on the remarks, photographs, or recordings they share. Time after time, they get malware: infections, phishing, smishing, worms, for example, Koobface, and different noxious code.

Informal community sites are a top focus of cyber criminals in light of the fact that the destinations are so lucrative. They exhibit colossal quantities of clients, and the clients are inclined to trust and react to the substance—tolerating welcomes, entering account or other private data, and tapping on connections. Lawbreakers misuse this trust to naturally take information, cash, or figuring assets.

A Protection Primer

Like web security by and large, online networking security is unpredictable and continually developing. You can illuminate yourself with assets, for example, http://tools.cisco.com/security/focus/home.x and http://socialmediasecurity.com/, and by checking the protection strategies of online networking locales.

For one thing, here are a few proposals for how a little business can guard itself.

1. Ensure that users frequently update their applications

Frequently redesign and fix the programs, antivirus programming, and online networking modules stacked on worker tablets, desktops, and PDAs. Likewise, redesign web applications, for example, Adobe® PDF Reader and Flash® Player, Apple QuickTime, Windows Media Player, RealPlayer, and JavaScript. Redesigns battle site threats, for example, SQL infusions.

2.   Build security into your network

Apply insurance composed particularly for the way you work together; your Value-Added Reseller (VAR) accomplice can offer you some assistance with determining the best devices and designs. The perfect devices disentangle the utilization of multilayer security advancements that offer assurance both inside and past your system border; here are some that are evaluated for little organizations:

- *Security machines*, for example, the Cisco SA 500 Series Security Appliances join a firewall and more far reaching security in one easy to-oversee box. For instance, they can coordinate Cisco cloud-based email and web security and also the interruption counteractive action framework (IPS) programming. For organizations that require more granular control or administrative consistence, Cisco ASA 5500 Series Adaptive Security Appliances can dissect and report activity down to the parcel level.
- *IPS* programming can consequently identify and obstruct certain sorts of system associations or movement, for example, shared and texting((IM). Also, if outside aggressors sneak past your firewall, the IPS can keep them from increasing further.
- *Hosted administrations* offer assurance straightforwardly "through the cloud". For instance, Cisco ProtectLink Gateway works at your system's Internet passage point to evaluate the notoriety of every site that representatives visit, square undesired sites, and progressively channel substance and email. Cisco ProtectLink Endpoint concentrates on shielding PCs from malware, and can keep PCs without upgrading security from getting to the Internet.
- *Routers*, for example, Cisco Small Business Routers have a fundamental firewall worked in; most likewise backing the Cisco ProtectLink Gateway administration.

3.   Block or limit employee access to sites

Most representatives anticipate that their working environment will give Internet administration. Yet their own long range informal communication can gobble up profitability and transmission capacity.

One safeguard is to boycott utilization by and large. A more sensible methodology is to control what sorts of destinations can be gotten to, and when. For instance, you could utilize Cisco ProtectLink Gateway to bind informal community site access to lunchtime.

4.   Educate employees and create a use policy

The Security's special case is human conduct. To guard against information spillage and malware, set up an organization approach and teach representatives on their obligations. The key messages for person to person communication destinations are:

- Customize; never default. Reset the default protection settings on your records to control who can see what, how your data can be sought, and which applications you'll empower (news sustains? Connections to advertisements?).
- Be a slippery target. Make a special secret key for every site, make every watchword solid, and change it each 90 to 120 days. Think about utilizing as a secret word administration arrangement.
- Post content prudently. Try not to share anything that you wouldn't need seen by any individual from people in general, including a contender, financial specialist, or potential boss. Battle data fraud: Never offer private data to anybody through long range informal communication.
- Develop an online networking, security arrangement and incorporate it in your organization's worthy use strategy for PCs. You can discover a few cases at SANS, Social Media, Business Council, and Cisco.

The approach structure needs to consider the accompanying significant security ideas when managing an outside application:

- Social media is for the most part in view of outsider "cloud" applications and, consequently, your organization can't control their security.
- Social media web applications and downloadable applications have the same security challenges as all other online applications and other introduced programming applications.
- The overall population is as included with your organization's utilization of online networking as you may be, and your strategy needs to offer direction to your workers on the most proficient method to handle open collaborations.
- Your organization ought to have an open adaptation of your online networking approach that clarifies your positions on social networking.

Sharing of information is an absolute necessity in online networking, yet information sharing is likewise a key part of assaults from both a mechanical hacking viewpoint and in addition a substantial point of view.

- The Malicious code is simpler to share by means of online networking entries and downloadable applications that can then interface back to the professional workplace to present infections, Trojans, and other malware.

- Reputation administration is frequently more imperative than secure innovation based controls while tending to the dangers because of online networking.
- Enable encoded correspondences to the online networking website when conceivable. This is difficult with most locales, yet applications are accessible that can help with this errand. One sample is HTTPS all over the place from the Electronic Frontier Foundation (https://www.eff.org/https-all over the place).

Tip: Sites for following vulnerabilities incorporate National weakness Database, Security Database and Open Source helplessness Database. On these locales, you can hunt down innovations and online networking channels you use for any known vulnerabilities that may trade off your security.

HTTPS Everywhere is a Firefox expansion (conveyed as a planned exertion between The Tor Project and the Electronic Frontier Foundation). It scrambles your correspondences with different huge locales. Various districts on the Web offer some obliged support for encryption over HTTPS, yet make it difficult to use. For example, they may default to decoded HTTP, or fill mixed pages with associations that retreat to the decoded site. The HTTPS Everywhere expansion settles these issues by adjusting all sales to these destinations to HTTPS.

When you present the HTTPS Everywhere add-on in Firefox, it qualities encryption on the destinations it covers.

HTTPS Everywhere really offers insurance against Firesheep and the product at present backings different destinations, for example, Google Search, Wikipedia, bit.ly, GMX, and Wordpress.com web journals, and, obviously, Facebook and Twitter. As Facebook and Google and different locales make HTTPS associations all the more promptly open and a default alternative, the risk of decoded interchanges will diminish.

The following are ways to minimize risks in social networks:

- You ought to just distribute data that you are consummately OK with, contingent upon what you need to achieve.
- Add just individuals you trust to your contact list.
- Avoid clicking surprising connections originating from individuals you don't have the foggiest idea.
- Never completely believe anybody you don't have a clue about that well.

A New Dynamic, Mobile, Flexible Architecture

At the point when most business was "neighborhood", most security was area driven. Area driven security will be security that depends fundamentally on the area of a system gadget to settle on security implementation choices. In this way, in the event that you have a firewall that characterizes a "border," security choices are made by the firewall in light of whether a gadget is "inside" or "outside" the edge. Basically, the choices depend on the doled out IP address and system subnet of the gadget. That functions admirably when clients have a solitary gadget that doesn't move much (a desktop), in a settled base. After some time, security groups have extended this model to layer progressively more "trusted" edges more profound and more profound into the system. In this way, you have 3-level application designs, where the "center" of the application is inside of the deepest edge and layers of security structure progressive concentric circles around the center. This research work is documented in the work of Andreas M. Antonopoulos (2011)

Layered security and resistance inside and out are not broken in essence. Maybe it is static layers and static borders that are broken. The impediments of this model get to be clear when you attempt to move a gadget, either a server (e.g. VMotion or livemigration), or a customer (a cell phone). At the point when versatility is presented, the engineering of concentric layers of security rather turns into a hindrance to change. To settle that, security groups regularly turn to network contrivances, such as punching gaps through firewalls, utilizing VLANs and VPNs to connection

Figure 2. Dynamic, flexible security architecture

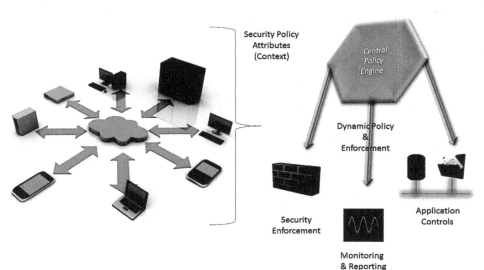

security "zones" and always showing signs of change firewall tenets to adjust to new applications. The reason security groups resort to "kludgy" arrangements is on account of mapping a dynamic arrangement of clients and applications to static and area based security design is incomprehensible. Definitely the framework turns out to be excessively mind boggling, making it impossible to oversee.

Today's dynamic, versatile and adaptable organizations require similarly rapid, adaptable and portable security. The security display that accomplishes this is a character driven model that is area free, for client and application recognizable proof. In such a model, security controls are connected construct basically in light of whom you are not where you are in the system. Area can be mulled over, obviously, yet it is stand out of the characteristics considered by the security strategy. The most imperative trait is the client character, which turns into the key strategy part to control access to applications and the framework. Client character is likewise basic to logging, checking and review works that can be utilized to track who access what and when, for administrative consistence or strategy reasons.

A personality driven foundation comprises of 3 noteworthy design segments: endpoints, approach authorization focuses, and strategy choice focuses. The center of the engineering is a strategy motor (the approach choice point) that permits focal administration of the client driven arrangements for the business. The arrangement motor is the place strategy choices are made by looking at characteristics, (for example, client personality, gadget sort, area, time of day, application and so forth.) to element access strategies.

As a sample, a strategy might express that a particular gathering of clients (e.g. attendants) can get to a particular application (e.g. tolerant records) from particular stations, at particular times, over particular systems. By concentrating approach administration, the strategy motor permits organizations to apply a reliable arrangement over their whole system and notwithstanding growing to include outside (e.g. SaaS) applications.

The other two parts of dynamic, versatile, and adaptable security design are the endpoints and the implementation focuses. Endpoints are the end client gadgets, additionally applications, databases, servers, and different gadgets associated with the system. Requirement focuses are different security gadgets or system gadgets (switches, switches, and so forth.) that can authorize access control choices. While implementation is dispersed over the system, strategy is incorporated in an arrangement motor. Centralization of strategy means security groups can adjust strategies in one spot and quickly present new applications, new legitimate zones and trust zones, new gadgets and new business forms. Since authorization is conveyed, gadgets can move from system fragment to network section, bouncing from wired to remote to portable remote systems while keeping up reliable access approaches and application experience.

Moving from Location-Centric to Identity-Centric Security

On the off chance that you need to move from area driven to character driven security, you should change the way you assess and purchase security arrangements. To guarantee you are purchasing an answer that consolidates personality driven standards.

Here are some key inquiries:

- What is the essential security trait in access control arrangements (is it IP location or client?)
- Does the security arrangement permit focal control of approaches for all systems (wired, remote LAN, versatile remote, remote/VPN)
- Can a client move from system to arrange, under the same approach (or do you have to characterize strategies in numerous spots)
- Can a server move without changing security strategy
- Can another application be included without rolling out improvements in requirement focuses (e.g. firewalls)
- Can a client's entrance be observed end-to-end on various gadgets paying little respect to IP address or system area?

CONCLUSION

Understanding the boundless group of risks is the essential step in ensuring satisfactory affirmation of sensitive data. All frameworks are vulnerable against cybersecurity threats. A complete data security framework is urgent for mitigating these threats and keeping a data break. A sweeping approach to manage data security starts with appreciation the framework, its building, customer people, and mission necessities. Case in point, security threats for frameworks with significant customer masses and frameworks connected with the web are particularly high. Once the risks have been assessed and various leveled security game plans decided, security designing should be arranged and a security course of action executed. Enduring utilization of the security game plan will reduce shortcoming to advanced threats and extension the general security of an affiliation's data.

Static security designs are hindering your exceedingly dynamic, portable and interconnected business. Security might go about as a hindrance to your business' advancement, innovation reception and intensity. More security spending won't settle the essential crisscross between security that is area driven and business that endeavors to work anyplace, at whatever time, on any gadget. You should begin arranging a move to character driven, setting mindfulness and dynamic security taking into account a design that brings together strategy and circulates authorization. At exactly that point can your clients be freed to be gainful and team up without obstructions, expanding your organization's rate of progress, advancement and rivalry.

At the point when utilizing private online networking accounts:

- Carefully consider the sort and measure of data you present with respect to on your work obligations. Try not to post data that is not for open discharge from your present or past employment parts.
- Restrict the measure of individual data put on online networking sites. Abstain from posting data, for example, your home or business locale, telephone numbers, spot of work and other individual data that can be utilized to target you.
- Monitor the data companions and partners post about you to keep the unapproved divulgence of your own data.
- Consider restricting access to presented individual information on 'companions as it were'.
- Apply any accessible security and protection alternatives to your records and utilize a "private" profile where relevant.
- Use an individual email address as opposed to an official email address while making individual profiles, and utilize a nom de plume instead of unveiling your full name. In the event that conceivable, make your email address private to those survey your page.
- Several online networking sites permit clients to 'quit' of permitting internet searchers to hunt and show your data. In the event that conceivable, utilize this 'quit' highlight.
- Review the site security and protection arrangements frequently, as these can change with negligible correspondence to clients.
- Be careful about getting to obscure site connections or connections, spontaneous contact and tricks, (for example, using fake profiles).
- Report any suspected security occurrences when you or a partner has posted touchy or characterized data on online networking sites to your defensive security group. Report any suspicious contact made to you or a partner through online networking sites.

REFERENCES

Ahlqvist, T., Bäck, A., Halonen, M., & Heinonen, S. (2008). Social media road maps exploring the futures triggered by social media. *VTT Tiedotteita - Valtion Teknillinen Tutkimuskeskus,* (2454), 13.

F., C. (n.d.). Global Information Policymaking and Domestic Law. *Indiana Journal of Global Legal Studies,* 467-487.

Guide to Data Protection. (n.d.). Retrieved from https://ico.org.uk/for-organisations/guide-to-data-protection/

KEY TERMS AND DEFINITIONS

Blogs: Are the websites, independently by bloggers. Here, content with dated items are arranged in reverse chronological order.

Browser: Is a tool to view websites. It is also used to get all the content accessible there onscreen or by downloading.

Cloud Computing: As per definition by NIST (USA), Cloud Computing is defined as "a model for enabling convenient, on-demand network access to a shared pool of configurable computing resources (e.g., networks, servers, storage, applications, and services) that can be rapidly provisioned and released with minimal management effort or service provider interaction".

Comment: Is provided by blogs to the readers to include comment under items. It might also provide feed for comment.

Content: Is a text, image, video or any other helpful material on the Internet.

The Forum: Is a debate area in which where people can post messages or comment on existing messages independently of time/place.

Link: Is the highlighted text or image which allows you to jump from one web page/content to another when clicked.

The Network: Is a organization containing nodes and interconnection between them. In social network nodes are people and links are the relationships between them.

Chapter 9
Trust, Privacy, Issues in Cloud–Based Healthcare Services

Shweta Kaushik
JIIT Noida, India

Charu Gandhi
JIIT Noida, India

ABSTRACT

In recent era individuals and organizations are migrating towards the cloud computing services to store and retrieve the data or services. However, they have less confidence on cloud as all the task are handled by the service provider without any involvement of the data owner. Cloud system provides features to the owner, to store their data on some remote locations and allow only authorized users to access the data according to the role, access capability or attribute they possess. Storing the personal health records on cloud server (third party) is a promising model for healthcare services to exchange information with the help of cloud provider. In this chapter, we highlight the various security issues and concerns such as trust, privacy and access control in cloud based healthcare system that needs to be known while storing the patient's information over a cloud system.

DOI: 10.4018/978-1-5225-1002-4.ch009

INTRODUCTION

Utilization of most recent technology such as cloud computing in healthcare ser-vices provides a new direction for healthcare organizations to enhance the quality of service delivery, reduce the cost and make it efficient to be used by users belongs to different category. Popularity of healthcare services and cloud computing among users also make an increase in the demand of cloud based healthcare services. In addition, diseases are becoming more complex and new advancements in technology and research have facilitated the emergence of new and more effective diagnoses and treatment techniques (Singh, 2008). In the last few years, healthcare services have achieved many improvements from individual solutions to the organization level solution, and from a single individual system, which provides local and limited resolution to more interconnected ones, which provides incorporated and broad resolution for a particular diagnosis problem. Complexity of cloud based healthcare services also improve from passive and reactive system to active and interconnected systems, which mainly focuses on the quality of the system. Use of cloud in healthcare services also introduces the use of advance technology such as improved database system to provide a reliable solution. Cloud computing will also reduce the burden of healthcare services by introduction of service provider who is completely responsible for managing the complex data of different health-care services and handling all the users queries which reduce the maintenance and operational cost of such a large system, as the same system is required by multiple healthcare organization so the service provider needs to setup one system which can be used by multiple organizations and so the cost can be divided among the organizations. Use of cloud computing also opened a new opportunity window for healthcare services to use and share their data with organizations and users such as researchers, doctors, hospitals, organizations like WHO etc. that will be helpful for introduction of new technique or improve the quality of existing techniques of any healthcare services. But this sharing of patient's data will not come alone, it also introduce the new security challenges that needs to be handled. Strict rules and regulations while sharing of patient's data is necessary to maintain its privacy such as who is going to use the data, what amount of critical information accessed by a particular user etc. Dealing with security and privacy of any confidential data which is shared over the network, introduces several threats such as exposure of patient's sensitive data, selling of the secret information of patient by a service provider to other service provider(s). Once an individual or organization stores the healthcare information over the cloud system they do not have any physical possession on it and cannot figure out that which information is sold or distributed to other users and what are the various securities needs to be concerned by that particular service provider. In this chapter, we understand the various privacy and security issues come into picture when integrate cloud computing with healthcare services and how to maintain trust between different communicating parties to develop an efficient and sound system. In addition, we also discuss the benefits and limitations of cloud based healthcare services with strategic recommendation for the adoption of cloud computing in healthcare services.

CLOUD BASED HEALTHCARE SERVICES CHALLENGES/ ISSUES

Although the cloud based healthcare service provide several benefits to various users such as healthcare industry, researchers, medical clinics and doctors, but also come with various challenges of cloud computing and e-healthcare services. These challenges require more attention as the system is storing, transferring and processing the very confidential and sensitive data of different patients. It increases the challenges for data storage and its maintenance because if the system is not secure than no user will store or retrieve the data. Various challenges specific to a cloud based health care system are broadly divided into two categories as (i) Technical (Momtahan, 2007) and (ii) Non- technical (Momtahan, 2007) challenges as shown in Figure 1, which are further summarized below as:

Figure 1. Cloud based healthcare service issues

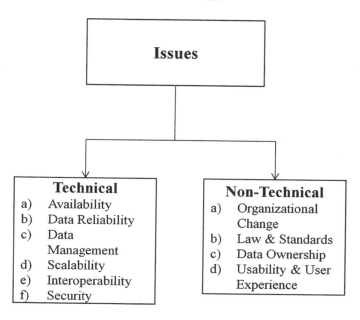

1. **Technical Challenges:** Introduction of new technique in existing technique will never come alone. It also comes with new challenges for its proper adoption and utilization in the existing techniques. Similarly, integration of cloud and healthcare services also come with new challenges, to be solved before adoption of cloud by any individual or organization. Some of the technical challenges as shown in Figure 1, in cloud based healthcare services are summarized as:

    a. **Availability:** Data and service availability is a crucial requirement for every healthcare service provider as without any data/service availability there is nothing to operate. Cloud based healthcare service providers must ensure that data/ service required by the users is available for 24 x 7 without any interruption or degradation in service performance. Since, cloud data is stored at the remote server which may be lost due to software failure, hardware failure, network failure etc, it is necessary to take the data backup and replicate it at multiple locations. This ensures the continuity of services as per the user's requirements even after the loss of data. In addition to this, hardware and software upgrade, reconfiguration and installation should also not interrupt the healthcare services.

    b. **Data Reliability:** In cloud based system, data will come from various remote locations which increase the chances of corrupt and incorrect data. To handle this problem, it is provider's responsibility to provide consistent and error-free data constantly without any disturbance due to hardware and software failure. Service provider always need to make sure that data replicated at different locations is consistent and follows the ACID (Atomicity, Consistency, Integrity, and Durability) property during any transaction.

    c. **Data Management:** In cloud based healthcare services huge amount of patient's information is stored at server site which may include some confidential data as well. There is need for secure data storage and its maintenance against any security fault occurs in public cloud. Delivery and processing of confidential data also required some security concerns for its efficient and scalable delivery to the user according to the security measure defined.

    d. **Scalability:** Cloud stores the medical data for millions of patient at different healthcare service providers which requires the scalability of cloud to handle increasing data in a skilled manner. In the cloud based system, this can be increased by increasing the capability of various service nodes such as network connections; efficient operational and management storage units. Scalability requires dynamic configuration and reconfiguration as well as an automatic resizing of used virtualized hardware resources (Vaquero, 2008).

e. **Interoperability:** Cloud based healthcare services are provided not from a single service provider instead different service providers are responsible for handling different types of data of a single patient. For example, one service provider may store highly resolution medical images of a patient while other one is responsible for storing its personal information, lab reports, prescription, and medical history. There is a requirement for interoperability which requires defining some open source API/ protocol or agreed framework between different service providers to achieve integrity and presence of different servers at the same time. A good interpolation system also facilitates an efficient migration between different service providers to access the required data. One of the prominent solutions for this is to utilize the concept of Service-oriented Architecture (SOA) (Al-Jaroodi, 2012) for cloud based healthcare services. SOA allows the services to be easily accessible and available as per users need using standardized protocol without considering the infrastructure, implementation, development or deployment model.

f. **Security:** Since, in cloud based healthcare services, the data is stored and retrieved from remote location without any physical access of the data owner and provided by number of service provider, requires the security concern regarding its storage, access control, integrity, confidentiality etc. It is a prime feature to provide secure and adequate access control and authentication management while transferring the data from service provider to users. In addition to this, there is also a requirement to store the data in encrypted format at the service provider's end to protect it from any malicious activity and vulnerability by any adversary or service provider to get the exact data. There are several mechanisms to impose high security, but requires high computation complexity and cost which make them inefficient for cloud based system.

2. **Non-Technical Challenges:** Apart from the technical challenges there are some non-technical challenges come in picture with the adoption of cloud in healthcare services which requires high concerns for its proper utilization and adaption by individual and organization. The various non-technical challenges as shown in Figure 1 are summarized as:

a. **Organizational Change:** Use of cloud in healthcare services brings many important changes in the field of research, organization boundaries, medical treatments and business processes. Cloud based healthcare services introduce new workflow of business process as all the documentation and medical records are stored, retrieved, and processed at the cloud. It requires the businesses and organizations to be updated as per the cloud storage and deliverance for its confidential data storage and accessibility according to defined security policies without any physical introduction of owner for its maintainability.

b. **Law & Standards:** There is no adequate definition for the law and standards to be followed for the cloud based healthcare services for any technical, clinical or business practices. It will bring new security requirements such as interoperability, data transmission, policies etc. Currently, some guidelines are defined for healthcare system which can be utilized by the cloud system to provide e-healthcare services. For example, the Systematized Nomenclature of Medicine (SNOMED) drafts a new layout for medicines for the purpose of storing and/ or retrieving records of any medical concern (Cote, 1986). Another example is World Health Organization (WHO) issued the International Classification of Diseases tenth revision (ICD-10) which specify the special coding for complaints, diseases, external reason for injury and sign of abnormal findings`.

c. **Data Ownership:** There are no proper guidelines define for ownership of data in healthcare systems. As data of any patient can be claimed by patient itself, doctor who treat the patient and hospital or clinic which provide the medical treatment for that particular patient. This challenge needs to be highly concern to draw proper guidelines and policies when storing any patient record over cloud based services.

d. **Usability & End Users Experiences:** This challenge concerns for the data usage, access and storage at the cloud based healthcare services by the various users. There are different type of users exists who try to access their required data from the cloud, which requires the proper authentication and access control pre-implementation to provide the data to the users according to their usability and experiences.

LIMITATION FOR CLOUD BASED HEALTHCARE SERVICES

• **Implementation and Maintenance Cost:** Integration of healthcare services with cloud computing requires a lot of cost for its implementation and maintenance especially in small and medium sized organizations. The investment in hardware, software and technical infrastructure with healthcare services implementation is a time consuming process as it requires to maintain lots of data about many patients, doctors etc. In addition to this a well-qualified and dedicated team with proper funding is required for a regular day-to-day data management and maintenance activities.

- **Fragmentation and Insufficient Exchange:** In most healthcare systems separate administrative systems exist for the different departments of healthcare service provider. It stores the patient data in dispersed manner where certain part of information is associated with only restricted department, some associated with clinical purpose and some of the information available publically. All departments have their own way to store the data. This dispersal of patient data at several locations with their different storage brings a new challenge to combine the complete information about a particular patient and share it at different cloud based healthcare service providers.
- **Lack of Regulation:** There are no well-defined and established laws for the patient record communication between two communicating parties for its privacy maintenance. There is a high requirement to define the various rules and regulation for sharing of patient's personal health records at different level of user access, organizations and countries to maintain the security and privacy and protect the patient personal health record from any malicious activity.
- **Lack of Cloud Deployment Model:** There are no well-defined standards for cloud based healthcare service provider to build an effective and efficient system. It consists of data types for data storage, in which form data is stored, its usage, security protocols for its data access and storage, how to obtain data and at which time frequency a new data will be capture. Apart from these challenges a biggest challenge is to develop and maintain a multidimensional system.

TRUST IN CLOUD BASED HEALTHCARE SERVICES

Trust means a faith, confidence of doing a job as expected without introducing any vulnerability while performing any task. 'An entity A is considered to trust another entity B when entity A believes that entity B will behave exactly as expected and required'' (ITU, 2009). Trust can incorporate security by performing validity of its performance, loyalty, encoding data and user-friendliness to attract other towards it. In cloud based healthcare services, patient's data is stored at cloud provider and user will get the required data from cloud provider also. There is a need arise for a mutual trust between various communicating parties to ensure that data stored and retrieved from cloud is intact without any malicious activity done during data transformation. Data owner requires that the service provider should be trustworthy to store its confidential data without any exposure to unauthorized user and other service providers. On the other hand, users who will retrieve its data from the service provider also require that provider is trustworthy, who deliver the exact correct data without any loss of integrity and damage of data. Thus, trust plays a vital role in cloud based healthcare services as it stores the patient's sensitive data which is delivered to other users such as hospitals, researchers, medical clinics, pharmacies etc. in intact form. If there is no trust maintain between different communicating parties than patient will not store it's confidential and essential data for other users, over the cloud based healthcare services provider. One of the prominent solutions for trust maintenance between different communicating parties is Service Level Agreement (SLA) signed between them and another one is the inclusion of Trusted Third Party (TTP). This TTP is responsible for auditing the data stored at service provider either periodically or dynamically and report to data owner if any misbehavior found. Thus, the entire users and data owner relying on TTP for secure and efficient transactions as the malicious activities can be caught by TTP.

TRUST MECHANISMS IN CLOUD HEALTHCARE SERVICES

Broadly, trust can be classified based on trustor's anticipation as (Huang, 2013): 1) Trust in performance- is what the trustee performs and 2) Trust in belief - is what the trustee believes. Based upon these, various trust mechanisms are defined for defining the trust between different communicating parties, which are summarized as shown in Figure 2.

Figure 2. Trust mechanisms

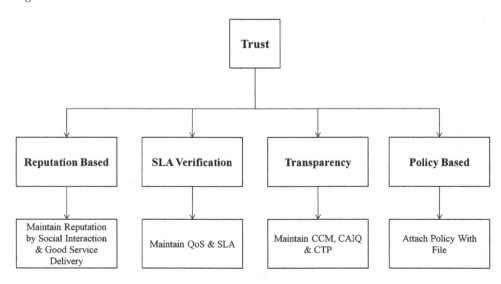

Reputation Based Trust

Reputation and trust are two different things but are related. Knowing the reputation of an entity, other entities can trust it but, having trust on an entity will not play any role to its reputation. Reputation based trust mechanism is broadly used in the area of P2P network and e-commerce. Reputation of any web service can be calculated by its collective analysis of feedback or opinions taken from different users on the basis of different aspect of service performance. The reputation of any cloud healthcare service or service provider will undoubtedly impact the choice of user for that particular service or service provider. Therefore, cloud based healthcare service provider needs to construct and maintain higher reputation. Usually, any web service which has high reputation is highly trusted by the most users. In cloud based healthcare services user first make a comparison of various service provider according to its reputation and then store and retrieve confidential data only on/from the service provider which has high rating given by the other entities without requiring any additional knowledge. At the initial stage, there is belief but afterward based on the performance of service delivered trust is maintain.

SLA Verification Based Trust

SLA (Service Level Agreement) is a legal contract signed between the different communicating parties in cloud based system. User (generally patient) stores the highly sensitive data on cloud, only if there is a proper contract signed for security and QoS maintenance assurance. On the other hand, different users (doctors, researchers, medical clinic, pharmacy etc.) will retrieve the data from service provider after establishing an initial trust and verifying the agreement signed between users and service provider regularly. Many SLA based trust models have been proposed (Haq, 2013,Pawar, 2012). Trust with verification is a best option for the fine relationship between the different communicating parties. Major issue with SLA is that user focuses only on visible components (such as GUI) of service provider while invisible components such as security and privacy issues are generally missed. Also user can not monitor QoS and SLA verification at their end because of less capability and require lots of computation and time requirements. Due to this a need for TTP arises to handle these entire tasks for data owner and user.

Transparency Based Trust

Transparency in the service user by the user creates a high trust and belief between the various parties for accessing the correct service without any discrepancy. To sustain and enhance the transparency of service provided by the service provider to the users Cloud Security Alliance (CSA) introduces the "Security, Trust and Assurance Registry (STAR)" program (CSA 2011). This program allows the service providers to circulate their self-impression of security control measures, in either "Cloud Control Matrix (CCM)" or "Consensus Assessments Initiatives Questionnaire (CAIQ)" form. Here, CCM is a cloud model which outlines the alignment of service provider with CSA security guide. CAIQ contains several questions which cloud users or auditor may ask to verify the transparency of service. Apart from this CSA also adopts Cloud Trust Protocol (CTP). This is a request-response mechanism used by the users for the confirmation of cloud provider transparency. The main aim of CTP with transparency is to generate an evidence- based assurance to check that everything is done in the same way as required without any vulnerability. Therefore, in cloud based healthcare services, data owner or user first check the transparency of the services provided by the service provider using one of the mechanisms i.e. CCM, CAIQ or CTP to establish trust and on the basis of that store or retrieve data.

Policy Based Trust

In earlier approaches a formal mechanism was defined for trust between different communicating parties in cloud system. In addition to this, Public Key Infrastructure (PKI) is also widely used to maintain trust by employing the digital signatures, key/ attribute certification and validation. To ensure that data retrieved / stored from/on service provider's end is intact a policy is defined which contains the access criteria associated with the data and its corresponding key / attribute. Only the user who has the valid set of key/attribute can access the data. Similarly, in cloud based healthcare services only the user who meets certain aspect or policy as mentioned by the owner can only store the data. To simplify this, consider the example as shown in figure 3. Suppose a doctor associated with hospital A retrieve some data from healthcare service provider supposedly after satisfying the policy P1="(profession=doctor) $\wedge$(specialty = cancer treatment)$\wedge$(organization = hospital A)", which is signed by a patient using his private key K_p and also attach a certificate with some policy assigned to the data. Since doctor has all the attributes required to access the data, he can only decrypt the received data using patient's public key and attribute the doctor possess and verify the integrity of data using the digital signature.

Attribute Based Trust

Like, policy based trust approach attribute based trust is also an informal approach for establishing the trust between different communicating parties. Here, only the users who have required set of attributes with satisfying values can retrieve the data. In general form, we can formalize the attribute based trust as follows: believe(A,

Figure 3. Attribute hierarchy for data access

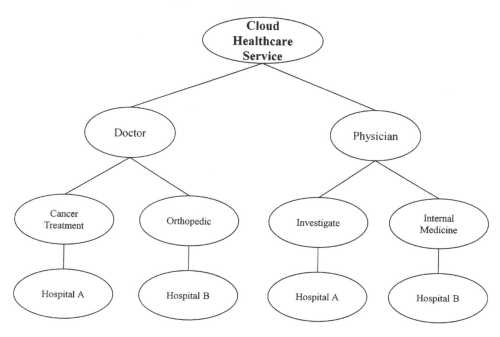

attr$_1$(x,v$_1$)) &....&(believe(A,att$_n$(x,v$_n$)) = trust(A,x,c) [Huang, 2013], which states that, if a user A believes subjects s has attribute att$_1$,att$_2$...att$_n$ with values v$_1$,v$_2$......... v$_n$ respectively. Than A can trust x performance and or data created/ delivered under specific situation c. Different cloud data owner may have their own different trust policies which involve different attributes for trust building. A common model sustains different attribute based trust using different policies for different users. The interrelation between policies based and attributes based relation is that, belief of a user to confirm a policy has a set of attribute with specified values for that particular policy.

As seen in Figure 4, trust of any entity in a cloud based system depends on several resources and other entities. A data owner can trust cloud provider for secure data storage using SLA based trust. A data owner can trust user by providing policy for trust. A data owner can trust auditor for its correct auditing by transparency based trust mechanism. Similarly, a user can trust cloud provider and cloud broker for correct delivery of required data/ service according to its reputation and SLA signed between them. Cloud broker, plays an important role in cloud system as the cloud broker is responsible for the conciliation between cloud users and service providers for the use of different services. The judgment of trust of various cloud entities depends on several attributes, as described in (Huang, 2013), which are shown in Figure 5.

Figure 4. Trust relation chain in healthcare services

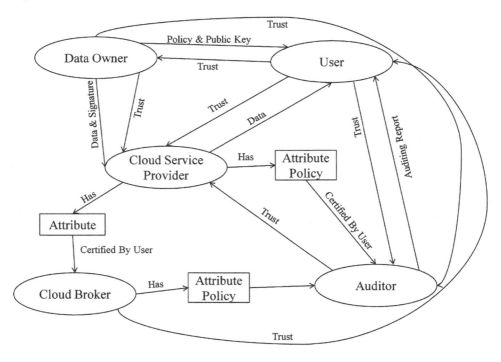

Figure 5. Judgment of cloud entities

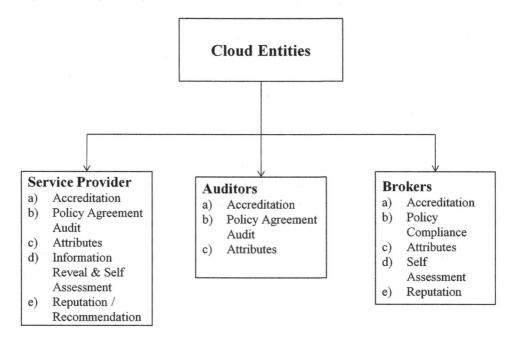

SECURITY AND PRIVACY REQUIREMENTS IN CLOUD BASED HEALTHCARE SERVICES

Privacy

Privacy means to keep the data secret and hide from unauthorized access. Privacy of data can be obtained by encoding, encryption, translations of data, which transforms the confidential data into some other form. It generally includes protection of data from any malicious activity by the adversary. In cloud based healthcare service, patient's information is stored which may include some sensitive information also. Users can access the data according to defined role, access criteria or attribute assigned to them. Data owner requires that service provider will deliver its data according to the access criteria defined by him in order to protect the data from unauthorized access. Since data owner can not completely trust service provider for its data privacy so he can encrypt the data before outsource.

Security Issues

Apart from privacy and trust maintenance between different parties there are another security issues need to be considered i.e. authorization and access control, integrity, non- repudiation, network security, confidentiality. To provide the authorization and access control data owner can decide one of three mechanisms i.e., role based access control, user based access control or attribute based access control to allow the users to get required data. Owner also needs to notify service provider about access control for verification purpose before transferring the data to users according to their request. To prove that data integrity is maintained without any vulnerabilities owner can encrypt the data with digital signature. Only the authorized users have verification key to check the integrity of received data from the service provider to ensure that retrieved data is intact. As the data owner shares the verification key with user only. Some of the security requirements with their description and possible solutions are shown below in Table 1. In addition to this, security issues in cloud based system also encompasses the threats and risks, as summarized below, which may come because of external or internal users. Adoption of healthcare services in cloud based system requires having knowledge of these security risks and threats and a defined way to handle these.

Table 1. Security requirements

Security Requirement	Description with solutions
Authentication and access control	To provide the patient's data to authorized users according to their access criteria, there is a need of identification system. This system will be able to differentiate between the authorized and unauthorized users and allow only authorized users to access the required data according to their access criteria such as role, capability, identification etc. defined by the owner for its data accessibility.
Confidentiality & Privacy	To guarantee the confidentiality and privacy the data needs to be encrypted first and digitally signed by data owner before transfer over cloud system. Only the authorized user having the decryption key can decrypt it to original data and use the verification key to check its consistency. Service provider is unaware of this decryption key and verification key.
Integrity	Data owner need to sign its data and only the authorized users has its verification key to check whether they got the exact or malicious data. It will help to preserve the consistency and accuracy of delivered data.
Auditing	It helps to maintain the interoperability feature in cloud based system. The malicious activity is monitored by auditor and auditing reports are sent to owner to alert him. Owner takes necessary action as required. Auditing can be done by the data owner itself or he can hire a trusted third party for this task.
Trust	This is required to belief that data is stored at right place and also retrieved correctly without introducing any vulnerability. It can be achieved by a contract signed between the different communicating parties such as service level agreement.
Non-repudiation	This is required to ensure that communicating party will not deny from accessing, storing or receiving the data. This can be implementing by using a timestamp, encryption or digital signature between the different communications done between different parties.

Cloud Attacks

In a cloud system attacks can be divided into four types i.e. random, weak, strong and sustain attack. Each of these attacks depends on whether the attack is successfully activated and not on the threats they may introduce.

- **Random Attack:** In this attack, attacker will use simple tools and techniques to find any vulnerable work by scanning the internet randomly. Their main concern here is to find valuable information by deploying some tools/ technique and without any authentication.
- **Weak Attack:** In this attack, the target is service provider, to breach its security wall. These types of attackers are semi-skilled but more advanced and try to get the confidential information from the service provider with the help of customize tools.
- **Strong Attack:** In this attack, attackers are highly skilled with well-financed condition. Their target is a particular user or application in cloud which will

be entirely exploit by them. Generally, this group is specialized to target any specific service.

- **Substantial Attack:** In this attack, attackers are highly advanced and motivated to spoil any target service or organization even without any detection of targeted organization or investigative organizations who are specialized in internet security. They possess a very good knowledge of the resources and great intelligence to respond upon detection of their attacks.

Cloud Risks

In cloud, with each delivery model risks are associated which depends on several factors such as security requirements, development model, information confidentiality and resource availability. In general, various security risks in cloud without any concern for delivery model are summarized in Table 2.

Since last few years' research on cloud based healthcare service is growing fast and many researchers have presented their different framework which try to handle all the security issues as stated above. The security in healthcare services involves lot of challenges, as described earlier, that need to be addressed while delivering

Table 2. Security risks

Risks	Description	Approach
Privileged user access	Cloud providers have all the data of owner, which may include sensitive information and has complete access to this. Provider is not trusted party, therefore, confidentiality and access control for privileged user access is required to secure the data from any malicious activity.	Encryption before outsource the data and enforce laws and regulations.
Data location and segregation	Owner of the data does not have information regarding its data storage. They have only contractual or regulatory obligation which increase the risk concern for its data leakage to other user or organization without its knowledge.	Virtualization and SLA management.
Data disposal	Deletion and disposal of owner data is a risk, especially where resources are dynamically issued to users based on their access criteria. The risk of data not being deleted from data stores, data replication storage and physical media as required may increase the risk within the cloud.	Ensure ACID property during transmission and use of media sanitization techniques as per agreement between owner and provider.
Regulatory compliance	Owner stores its confidential data over cloud which requires to be protected from unauthorized access of users and service providers. Owner requires maintaining the integrity of data by attaching a certification with this.	Auditing and certification
Assuring cloud security	User gets the data from service provider which is not trusted. Thus, there is a security requirement for data verification and auditing to confirm the correct delivery of data from provider.	Auditing and SLA management

the patient confidential and sensitive data over cloud. It is like a multipart maze which requires lot of attention and hurdles to be solved before reaching to an optimal solution. The comparative analysis for the work of various researchers according to their approach, advantages and disadvantages is summarized in Table 3.

Table 3. Comparative study of cloud based healthcare system

Scheme	Objective/Purpose	Approach/ Technique	Advantages	Disadvantages
Ambulatory electrocardiographic monitoring in clinical and domestic environments (Saldarriaga, 2013)	An android and iOS based mobile application is developed for ambulatory electrocardiographic monitoring. It is utilized by the medical personnel to use their smart phones to guide diagnose procedures efficiently and manage the daily activities interconnecting several zones.	To get the ECG information of a patient kardia Board is utilized and for transmission Bluetooth 4.0 interface OS smart phones are utilized. Android and Apple iOS bases phones are used.	Patients can upload and view their ECG data as per requirements. Doctors are able to receive ECG waveform data about any patient from their smart phones compare it with previous ECGs and provide the diagnosis to patient's problems.	This application can be used only on Android based or apple iOS smart phones.
Securing Personal Health Records in Cloud Computing: Patient-centric and Fine-grained Data Access Control in Multi-owner Settings (Li, 2010)	Securing the personal health records of multiple owners.	Patient-centric and Fine-grained data access control to secure the health record of patients in cloud computing.	Provide the features as user revocation, break-glass access and fine grained data accessibility policies.	It increases the computation time for data owner and also there is a risk of patient's private data exposure by owner.
Managing Wearable Sensor Data through Cloud Computing (Doukas, 2011).	A wearable – textile platform is developed which collects the patient's heartbeat and motion data and send this detail to cloud system and store. This cloud system is responsible for monitoring, processing and send the alert for health to patients.	Use the Google cloud service for data storage and processing and HTTP/HTTPS protocol for data exchange. Google Chart for data visualization. Java for developing cloud application. Bluetooth interface to send data to Android Smartphone. Arduino board as a wearable part	This developed platform helps the doctors to monitor their patient's health and patients to get Health alert. .	Did not consider patient's data privacy and use of Bluetooth interface, which is easy to handle and control by adversary.
Achieving secure, scalable and fine-grained data access control in cloud computing (Yu, 2010)	Secure personal health records of patient's, reduce the computation time for data owner for user administration and key distribution to various users.	Data owner the cloud provider to done all the computation tasks and user access control for him without disclosing data using some advanced techniques as Proxy Re-Encryption (PRE),Key-Policy Attribute- Based Encryption (KP-ABE), and lazy re-encryption.	Cloud service provider is not able to know the exact data and perform all the computation tasks for uses and owner which reduce their computation overhead and improver the scalability.	There is no mechanism is defined for emergency situations and also data access policy is limited.

continued on following page

Table 3. Continued

Scheme	Objective/Purpose	Approach/ Technique	Advantages	Disadvantages
Tackling cloud security issues and forensics model (Ahmed, 2010)	To ensure confidentially and privacy of electronic health records and track activities of cloud service provider for healthcare services in cloud environment.	This model supports the various mechanisms for data authentication, its access control, authorization and security against any nonvolatile information. To get any volatile information this model installs the forensic system on cloud systems.	To provide security against cyber crimes Computer Forensic Tools (CFT) provides digital evidence. Patient's medical data is kept safe from cloud service providers.	Use of CFT promises to track volatile actions; but it cannot physically stop volatile action by itself.
DACAR Platform for eHealth Services Cloud (Fan, 2011)	Develop a platform for secure services in e-Health Cloud.	Digital signature, access control, hashing, Single Point of Contact (SPoC), identity mapping, integrity check-sum, encryption and audit trial etc.	A complete secure platform which takes care of all the security aspects for a patient heath record management in cloud based system.	Comprehensive assessment in a real healthcare environment;
Privacy Engineering: Personal Health Records in Cloud Computing Environments (Kaletsch, 2011)	Whenever a referral is made a secure electronic health record (EHR) exchange is made possible.	Patient's confidential data is stored at only trusted environment such as the physicians' practices and all the data is encrypted and signed before any transmission done. This encrypted data can only be decrypted by specialist receiver.	For all documents to be transferred, suggested and provides secure encryption and signatures scheme for patient data security.	In this model no integration is defined for patient and patient-centric functions.
Co-Designing an Intelligent Doctors-Colleagues-Patients Social Network (Pirahandeh, 2012)	Develop a platform for Communication between specialists, clinics and patients.	Windows 7and 3 GHZ Core workstations and P2P Tester simulator.	Information sharing. Better Communication among doctors and patients. Better security as DCP is a private cloud system. Users can access their data using Internet, mobile phones.	No security algorithm is proposed and also no consideration for health alert system for patients.
Securing the E-Health Cloud (Lohr, 2010)	Provide secure platform for users when they will access e-Health Cloud.	Develop Trusted privacy domains (TVD) systems which are able to divide the execution environment in the end-user platform into separated domains that are isolated from each other.	Overcome limitations of security features within end user platforms; reduce security risks; Automatic management (transparent TVD establishment, key management and policy enforcement).	No scalability is defined and complex Hardware requirements

BENEFIT OF CLOUD BASED HEALTHCARE SERVICE

With the involvement of cloud computing in healthcare services many problems of patients, researchers, medical clinic, pharmacy and doctors can be resolved. As doctor can get its patient details from anywhere at any time and patient can get sufficient treatment without any delay. Researchers can get data easily from a single place without moving everywhere and struggling for collecting the different types of data. It can reduce the time for their research work and the outcome of the research such as medicine of any disease, new solutions can be implemented in time. With electronic health record management patient can also get the prescription detail for the same type of problems easily and get the information about the various hospitals, doctors etc. to be consult from a single end without facing any problems. Collaboration solution can also be made easily with cloud system which helps in the improvement of research and medical world. Cloud based healthcare system also maintain the healthcare exchange information to deal with any serious problems during natural phenomena.

- **Better Patient Care:** Using cloud based healthcare services a doctor can acquire the complete information about its patient history and treatment previously given to him at anywhere, anytime and provide the suitable treatment accordingly.
- **Reduced Cost:** This feature is best suitable for small and medium healthcare service providers. As they can easily obtain the advanced technology and treatment for any diagnosis without investment in initial setup and operational cost. In addition to this, using cloud computing it becomes easy to get any patient medical record globally without investing any money in exchanging this information.
- **Resource Scarcity Resolved:** Use of cloud computing resolve the IT resources shortage issues. It will help the healthcare services providers to use the remote medical services to provide primary services for patient treatments. It also helps the diagnosis specialist to provide their services remotely which can be used by the user to save time and reduce the need of specialist in case of emergency.
- **Better Quality:** As the patient's data is stored on the cloud and the doctor, researcher, hospital and healthcare organization acts as a user so the data can be utilized by them to improve the facilities and increase the patient's safety. Thus provides a better quality of services to the patient.
- **Research Support:** Cloud based healthcare services stores a huge amount of data regarding many patients, diseases and diagnosis which can be globally accessible. Using this information a researcher can get the complete knowl-

edge and can develop a new and improved version with less investment and time.

- **National Security:** The cloud based healthcare service enhances the capability to observe the increase of communicable diseases and/or other disease. So it helps in identifying growing disease, the region which is infected by the disease, the blueprint of the disease and the cause of its occurrence. The Cloud based healthcare service acts as a system that can be used to notify hospitals and organizations worldwide about any growing disease thus helps in national security.

- **Strategic Planning Support:** The cloud based healthcare service can be utilized by System architects in development, arrangement, scheduling and financial plan for healthcare services. The cloud based healthcare service can interact with each other to determine the requirement of doctors, nurse, helping staff, labs, equipment, operating rooms, patient beds, medicines etc. to optimize the existing healthcare services, setup new facilities in existing healthcare services and setup new the healthcare services.

- **Financial Operation Support:** Provides the ability to support all the financial operations between healthcare service providers and patients as cloud acts as a negotiator between them. Cloud is responsible for the entire task related to billing, approval and agreement process in between the communicating parties.

- **Facilitate Clinical Trials:** Data stored at service provider allows the researchers, pharmaceutical companies and medical institutions to get required information for the trials of new medicines. Cloud stored a huge amount of data in interconnected fashion which make it easy to get the patient's data related to specific case and try new clinical cases on them to provide a new solution.

- **Forming Registries**: The data which need to be stored and shared should follow a special registry specified for specific patient, diseases and diagnosis etc. For example a patient is targeted as either heart patient or cancer patient to store or retrieve data.

STRATEGIC APPROVAL FOR CLOUD BASED HEALTHCARE SERVICE

Use of cloud computing requires a coordinated and integrated approach. This approach is a fundamental description of how to utilize the cloud computing advantages in healthcare services by any healthcare service providers. These strategic approvals include the following tasks as stated below:

- Understand the patient's information sensitivity and its importance before moving towards cloud computing.
- Decision about which information required more security and what should be the access criteria.
- Explore different cloud models according to the information storage and find out the best one among them for workload.
- Develop a performance indicator for each strategy to determine the benefit of the strategy for any healthcare industry.
- Develop a complete patient record file and store it over the cloud system in encrypted form as cloud is not trusted. With this update the service provider about the access criteria as well.
- Users will acquire their requisite data from cloud system and also verify it to ensure its correctness.
- Scalability of data is prime concern as more patients' data can be feed into the system according to its popularity.
- Auditing of data is required to ensure the data is intact and deliver to the users as specified in access criteria without any modification or alteration.
- Portability of data is required to allow various users (patients, researchers, pharmacy and doctors) to retrieve the data and service at anywhere, anytime without any struggle.

Whenever, any health organization tries to move its services over the cloud system, it requires to make a strategic planning before actually moving towards building a new model. This planning requires determining the benefits, risks, capability of the new system and drawing a complete strategic plan for its sound implementation to make it more efficient than existing one. Many researchers have provided several guidelines and requirements that need to be considered for the strategic planning for the introduction of cloud computing in new work. Marks & Lozano (Marks, 2010) defines 9 stages for the adoption of cloud computing life cycle by users to build any cloud project. These 9 stages are proof of concept, strategy & roadmap, architecture & modeling, implementation planning, implementing the plan model, expansion, collaboration, maturity and integration of different activities.

The US Federal Health IT strategic plan (UDHHS, 2008), also introduce some strategic planning for the adoption of cloud computing which can be utilize by the government to implement a cloud based healthcare services project. This plan gives a leadership role to office of National Coordinator for Health Information Technology, for the development and national level implementation of a healthcare system using the IT services to improve the efficiency and quality of healthcare services. This plan is mainly concern with 2 goals: population health and patient focused healthcare system with the objectives of adoption, privacy and security, interoperability and collaborative governance. Each strategy is also further associated with an objective to implement and assessed it.

Beside above guidelines, (Kuo, 2011) propose a Healthcare Cloud Computing Strategic Planning (HC2SP) model which can be used by any healthcare industry to gain the knowledge regarding the strategy, resources allocation and direction before migrate to cloud based healthcare services. This model includes the 4 stages as (see Figure 6): identification, evaluation, action and follow up.

Stage 1: Identification. In this stage first we need to analyze the current position and significance of healthcare organization's services and determine the basic objective of improvements in these systems after receiving the request of patient's. To get this root cause, analysis method can be used to find the exact problems in existing healthcare services.

The identification of correct objective with its scope is a prime concern to present an effective and efficient system to the patient (user). In addition, these teams also need to define the quality indicators for their defined services with its use and purpose. This stage is basically provides the strategic planning team with well defined problems and services required by the patients at his end.

Figure 6. HC²SP model

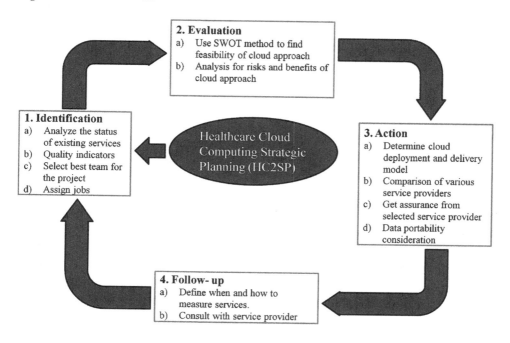

Stage 2: Evaluation. This stage deals with the evaluation of challenges and opportunities to be handle while adopting the cloud computing in healthcare services. To evaluate the risks and benefit for the adoption of cloud computing various evaluation strategies are defined in Cloud Security Alliance(Brunette, 2009), ENISA (ENISA, 2009) and NIST (Jansen, 2011)/ a patient/ user can also utilize the Strength, Weaknesses, opportunities and threats (SWOT) model to examine any cloud approach feasibility.

Stage 3: Action. After the evaluation of the new model, organization gets an idea whether it is feasible to go with the new model or not. If it is feasible than only organization moves towards the implementation step as stated below:

- Draw an idea about which type of cloud deployment and delivery model will be going to use.
- Make a comparison among various cloud provider according to their performance and reputation in the society.
- Select a best cloud provider among all after assuring the chosen one provides the security, privacy, quality of service as per the legal regulation and practices.
- Data portability, if required in future is easy to handle without any loss of data.

Stage 4: Follow- Up. After completing all the previous stages, the last task is to deploy the system and make a follow-up plan. This plan deals with measurement of the various services against specified indicators. If any discrepancy found, either from the user or provider prospective than resolve it at top priority. If the cloud service provider is not satisfying the service condition, than organization needs to either discuss the problems with service provider or migrate the data to another service provider for further processing.

DISCUSSION

It is clear that the cloud based healthcare service provides new promising direction for healthcare industry to move and succeed in this competitive world by introducing new advancement and experiments in existing one. It encompass the patient's data safety, reducing the operational cost, increase the popularity of healthcare services among the users, high computation and easy to access facility, maximum resources utilization, sharing of records, research support etc. In addition to this, sharing of knowledge and collaborate to introduce new medical services for all kind of diseases and provides diagnosis for them globally. As a result, cloud based healthcare services can be seen as potential solution for deliverance of high quality medical services at lower costs by healthcare providers. This integration of healthcare services and cloud computing provides many new IT solutions and advantages which may include:

- Allow multiple users such as doctors, patients, researchers to take benefit from this repository. Cloud store a huge amount of data which support medical research, enhance diagnosis, streamline process, administrative operation, financial support, resource abundance etc.
- It makes easy to exchange any medical information globally to enhance the medical activity and patient treatment using advance tools and techniques.
- Reducing the operation and maintenance cost of this integration results in all the related tasks are performed by the cloud providers.
- Increase the scalability, availability, flexibility and accessibility of healthcare information system.

However, these benefit not come alone. This integration also comes with the several security issues and challenges which need to be identified and resolved first before actually moving towards this new technology. The major concerns here are trust, privacy and security issues related to the patient's data which needs to be stored on cloud. The existing privacy and security measures introduce confidentiality, availability, authentication, access control etc. but it requires high computation with many loopholes. Since, patients store their sensitive/ confidential data over the cloud system. It reduces the high consideration for its data security regarding its accessibility, confidentiality, authenticity, auditing in order to provide a complete secure framework. In addition, there is proper care for various participants access criteria i.e, who can access the data and what amount of data it can access according to some predefined access criteria defined by the owner.

This collaboration of cloud and healthcare services also provides many feasible solutions for the distribution of responsibility and control among different users using trust maintenance between the communicating parties Trust is the prime concern that needs to be maintain between different community parties. Apart from these security concerns, some others challenges are also arise which require proper guidelines and standards need to be follow for the implementation and usage of cloud based healthcare services. These guidelines will handle the ability of data owners, user and service providers over the cloud system to maximize the cloud utilization with less investment cost. Many of these issues have been resolved and some needs to be resolved to obtain a sound system. To achieve this, there should be proper guidelines in this regards with suitable environment for development is required.

The cloud based healthcare services provides several benefit to small and medium healthcare industry and proves as a brilliant approach for them to utilize the latest technology with less operational cost. But, to make this possible in reality, there is a need of strong collaboration between the IT industry and research community to start their work in order to come up with an efficient and improve system. The system that handles all the issues and challenges that are faced by present cloud based healthcare services.

CONCLUSION

With the introduction of cloud computing in the field of healthcare service, a new direction is given to various users to communicate and share their required data from anywhere at any time and improve their practices and work. But, it also faces the various security concerns which need to deal carefully. In this chapter, we are dealing with the trust, privacy and various security issues in cloud based healthcare services and also provide the solutions to deal with any of these problems. In addition to this, we are also provides a brief description related to the benefit and strategic approval of cloud based healthcare services. Since patient's sensitive data is stored.on cloud based healthcare services which require high level of security and care. In future, a complete secure framework can be designed which handles all the security issues wisely and we have a mature system with every implementation and new version.

REFERENCES

Ahmed, S., & Raja, M. (2010, December). Tackling cloud security issues and forensics model. In High-Capacity Optical Networks and Enabling Technologies (HONET), 2010 (pp. 190-195). IEEE. doi:10.1109/HONET.2010.5715771

Al-Jaroodi, J., & Mohamed, N. (2012). Service-oriented middleware: A survey. *Journal of Network and Computer Applications*, *35*(1), 211–220. doi:10.1016/j. jnca.2011.07.013

Brunette, G., & Mogull, R. (2009). Security guidance for critical areas of focus in cloud computing v2. 1. *Cloud Security Alliance*, 1-76..

Cloud Security Alliance. (2011). *STAR (security, trust and assurance registry) program.* doi:10.1007/978-3-642-29852-3_7

Cote, R. A. (1986, October). Architecture of SNOMED: its contribution to medical language processing. In *Proceedings of the Annual Symposium on Computer Application in Medical Care* (p. 74). American Medical Informatics Association.

Doukas, C., & Maglogiannis, I. (2011, November). Managing wearable sensor data through cloud computing. In *Cloud Computing Technology and Science (CloudCom), 2011 IEEE Third International Conference on* (pp. 440-445). IEEE. doi:10.1109/CloudCom.2011.65

European Network and Information Security Agency. (2009). *Cloud Computing: Benefits, risks and recommendations for information security*. ENISA.

Fan, L., Buchanan, W., Thuemmler, C., Lo, O., Khedim, A., Uthmani, O., . . . Bell, D. (2011, July). DACAR platform for eHealth services cloud. In *Cloud Computing (CLOUD), 2011 IEEE International Conference on* (pp. 219-226). IEEE. doi:10.1109/CLOUD.2011.31

Haq, I. U., Alnemr, R., Paschke, A., Schikuta, E., Boley, H., & Meinel, C. (2010). Distributed trust management for validating sla choreographies. In Grids and service-oriented architectures for service level agreements (pp. 45-55). Springer US. doi:10.1007/978-1-4419-7320-7_5

Huang, J., & Nicol, D. M. (2013). Trust mechanisms for cloud computing. *Journal of Cloud Computing*, 2(1), 1–14.

Jansen, W., & Grance, T. (2011). Guidelines on security and privacy in public cloud computing. *NIST Special Publication, 800*(144), 10-11.

Kaletsch, A., & Sunyaev, A. (2011). *Privacy engineering: personal health records in cloud computing environments*. Academic Press.

Kuo, A. M. H., Borycki, E., Kushniruk, A., & Lee, T. S. (2011). A healthcare Lean Six Sigma System for postanesthesia care unit workflow improvement. *Quality Management in Health Care*, 20(1), 4–14. doi:10.1097/QMH.0b013e3182033791 PMID:21192203

Li, M., Yu, S., Ren, K., & Lou, W. (2010). Securing personal health records in cloud computing: Patient-centric and fine-grained data access control in multi-owner settings. In *Security and Privacy in Communication Networks* (pp. 89–106). Springer Berlin Heidelberg. doi:10.1007/978-3-642-16161-2_6

Löhr, H., Sadeghi, A. R., & Winandy, M. (2010, November). Securing the e-health cloud. In *Proceedings of the 1st ACM International Health Informatics Symposium* (pp. 220-229). ACM.

Löhr, H., Sadeghi, A.-R., & Winandy, M. (2010). Securing the e-health cloud. In *Proceedings of the 1st ACM International Health Informatics Symposium*. ACM.

Marks, E. A., & Lozano, B. (2010). *Executive's guide to cloud computing.* John Wiley and Sons.

Momtahan, L., Lloyd, S., & Simpson, A. (2007, June). Switched lightpaths for e-health applications: issues and challenges. In *Computer-Based Medical Systems, 2007. CBMS'07. Twentieth IEEE International Symposium on* (pp. 459-464). IEEE. doi:10.1109/CBMS.2007.104

Pawar, P. S., Rajarajan, M., Nair, S. K., & Zisman, A. (2012). *Trust model for optimized cloud services* (pp. 97–112). Trust Management, VI: Springer Berlin Heidelberg.

Pirahandeh, M., & Kim, D. H. (2012, April). Co-designing an intelligent doctors-colleagues-patients social network. In *Cloud Computing and Social Networking (ICCCSN), 2012 International Conference on* (pp. 1-4). IEEE. doi:10.1109/ICCCSN.2012.6215739

Recommendation, X. (2000). *509-The Directory: Public-key and attribute certificate frameworks.* International Telecommunication Union.

Saldarriaga, A. J., Pérez, J. J., Restrepo, J., & Bustamante, J. (2013, April). A mobile application for ambulatory electrocardiographic monitoring in clinical and domestic environments. In Health Care Exchanges (PAHCE), 2013 Pan American (pp. 1-4). IEEE. doi:10.1109/PAHCE.2013.6568306

Singh, H., Naik, A. D., Rao, R., & Petersen, L. A. (2008). Reducing diagnostic errors through effective communication: Harnessing the power of information technology. *Journal of General Internal Medicine, 23*(4), 489–494. doi:10.1007/s11606-007-0393-z PMID:18373151

US Department of Health and Human Services. (2008). *The ONC-Coordinated Federal Health IT Strategic Plan: 2008-2012.* US Department of Health and Human Services.

Vaquero, L. M., Rodero-Merino, L., Caceres, J., & Lindner, M. (2008). A break in the clouds: Towards a cloud definition. *Computer Communication Review, 39*(1), 50–55. doi:10.1145/1496091.1496100

World Health Organization. (2012). *International classification of diseases.* ICD.

Yu, S., Wang, C., Ren, K., & Lou, W. (2010, March). Achieving secure, scalable, and fine-grained data access control in cloud computing. In Infocom, 2010 proceedings IEEE (pp. 1-9). IEEE. doi:10.1109/INFCOM.2010.5462174

Chapter 10

A Methodological Evaluation of Crypto–Watermarking System for Medical Images

Anna Babu
M. G. University, India

Sonal Ayyappan
SCMS School of Engineering and Technology, India

ABSTRACT

Health care institution demands exchange of medical images of number of patients to sought opinions from different experts. In order to reduce storage and for secure transmission of the medical images, Crypto-Watermarking techniques are adopted. The system is considered to be combinations of encryption technique with watermarking or steganography means adopted for safe transfer of medical images along with embedding of optional medical information. The Digital Watermarking is the process of embedding data to multimedia content. This can be done in spatial as well as frequency domain of the cover image to be transmitted. The robustness against attacks is ensured while embedding the encrypted data into transform domain, the encrypted data can be any secret key for the content recovery or patient record or the image itself. This chapter presents basic aspects of crypto-watermarking technique, as an application. It gives a detailed assessment on different approaches of crypto-watermarking for secure transmission of medical images and elaborates a case study on it.

DOI: 10.4018/978-1-5225-1002-4.ch010

INTRODUCTION

Crypto-Watermarking is an evident area of research especially with the advent of medical related technologies. Health care institution demands exchange of medical images of number of patients to sought opinions from different experts. In order to facilitate storage and secure transmission of the medical images the applications related to telemedicine, transfer medical images by the aid of efficient crypto-watermarking system (Acharya, R., Bhat, P. S., Kumar, S., & Min, L. C, 2003). Since the transfer of medical imageries between hospitals and additionally among totally different consultants is common occurrence, the security and confidentiality of medical images is demanded. Crypto-watermarking helps in providing the appropriate information embedded in the medical images without creating an opportunity to defame an institution by rightful delivery of medical images to intended owner. The images can be protected while transmitting through channel when encryption is done. After the images get decrypted at the recipient side, it's prone to security breaches which can be protected by the use of watermarking. Thus crypto-watermarking is technique in which cryptography is combined with watermarking. In recent time, Crypto-watermarking techniques are gaining popularity as its finding importance in certain sensitive areas like healthcare, military communication and law-enforcement (Khan, A., Siddiqa, A., Munib, S., & Malik, S. A., 2014).

The utilization of internet for information spreads has created the vital call for security. Numerous robust encryption techniques for plain messages have been industrialized to fund this request. Privacy protection could be ensured with encryption and embedding the symmetric key in the encrypted domain. Encryption is the key for confidentiality and authentication of medical images transmitted. Encryption converts a data into unintelligible form. When an image with some secrecy need to be transmitted is encrypted, the provider unknown of the secret data tries to compress the encrypted image.

BACKGROUND

The Need for Crypto-Watermarking

The need for crypto-watermarking system is to give testimony concerning the security and confidentiality of images especially in sensitive areas like medical and military. In medical field the use of crypto-watermarking comes to play when the security of electronic patient records needs to be guaranteed along with privacy, authenticity and security of respective medical image. The regulations used for checking the protection of these data are the *Health Insurance Portability and Accountability*

Act (HIPAA) of US government and the European Data Protection Directive 95/46/ EC (Fernández-Alemán, J. L., Señor, I. C., Lozoya, P. Á. O., & Toval, A., 2013).

Crypto-Watermarking system has many applications which include the transfer of images whose security and confidentiality need to be verified also transfer of medical data for patients to undergo proper service regarding the health issues from various specialists. The use of crypto-watermarking in both areas is studied simultaneously in this chapter i.e. secure image transfer having details to preserve and secure electronic patient record transfer along with image. The medical data is protected by the aid of encryption and data hiding algorithms.

Medical field requires the transfer of medical data among practitioners for integrated checkups for patients around the globe. To aid these system EPR facilities for the hospital helps a lot for centralized access of patient records. EPRs give the opening for patients to take improved synchronized care from health providers and admission to their health material becomes easier. Electronic Patient Record (EPR) is a way to make things easier for all and to be better-quality informed and more involved in the patient's general health care. Providing EPRs among the different opinion collectors becomes critical with questions and apprehensions around the confidentiality and security of patient's condition information as well as hospitals fame.

Specific to protecting the information stored in EPRs, the HIPAA Security Rule of US government requires the health care providers to take up physical, administrative, and technical safeguards to protect a subject's electronic health information. Some safety measures that may be built in to EPR systems include:

In order to protect the data hold on in EPRs, the HIPAA Rule concerning security of US government needs the health care suppliers to take up physical, admin body, and technical safeguards to guard a subject's electronic health data. Some safety measures which will be in-built to EPR systems follow the mechanisms given below:

1. "Admittance controls mechanisms" like password keys and access PIN numbers, acts as a protective layer to limit access to one's confidential information's or limiting unauthorized access;
2. "Encryption" of information includes many patients health data cannot be easily interpreted or read except by authorized who can ˘decrypt" it, using a secret ``key" or any special type of key using symmetric or asymmetric methods;
3. "Review trail" which makes a note of who retrieved the info, what variations were completed and when.

The proposed method is motivated by the following observations: Next generation medical care technologies implies the need for security, confidentiality and privacy that will provide many benefits for health care delivery, but with advent of medical industry and its standards there are number of hindrances to privacy and security provisions that must be safeguarded in order to maintain basic virtuous principles in medical industry and its social existence (Zhang, X., 2011). Intention taken is to develop a technique that pools encryption of image and information (relevant data) hiding algorithm for benign transmission (Jaeger et al., 2014). Convenience of stream cipher motivates to use symmetric RC4 algorithm for EPR data encryption. The quick analysis and extraction of medical images and the relevant data also requires confidentiality to be preserved.

The chapter includes the transfer of image and EPR securely by the means of crypto –watermarking technique. Image is transferred securely after encryption by RC4. The secret key used for encryption by RC4 is in turn encrypted using a different technique - ElGamal crypto – system. Efficiency of this crypto -system is the major research paradigm in many works. The key encrypted by ElGamal is then entrenched in the image by the robust frequency DCT based – Spread spectrum watermarking approach. When EPR data needs to be embedded in the image it follows a different approach. The EPR security is other case study requirement for which different watermarking methodology is adopted based on size of data handled. When EPR is needed to be transmitted, the embedding algorithm can be differed as data varies considerably. Spatial pixel manipulations with research in area of Prediction – Error Domain is done for watermarking the EPR to images.

Thus case study in this chapter includes image encryption with secret key embedding with DCT based approach also EPR data embedding can be done in spatial prediction error domain using Rhombus prediction scheme as future scope. Analysis of results is done with quality metrics used as Peak Signal to Noise Ratio (PSNR) and Mean Square Error (MSE) values.

Image Encryption Techniques

Encryption is process of converting the message into a form that is illegible for any unauthorized personnel unless the key to decode the message is obtained which is only present with the authorized user. So it confirms the properties of authentication, integrity and confidentiality. Encryption can be based on *symmetric key encryption* and *public key encryption* scheme that can be applied to streams or blocks. Stream cipher is faster compared to block cipher methods. The keys used for encryption can be secret key, public-private key and shared key. RC4 is an example of stream cipher algorithm based on a symmetric secret key, RSA is an example of public-private key scheme, and Diffie Hellman key algorithm is worked upon shared secret key.

The encryption practice can be asymmetric, symmetric or hybrid. It can be functional to *blocks* or *streams*. The block encryption scheme applied to images, can meet with basically three inconveniences. The first and foremost one is when there is encryption of identical zones, they are found to be similar. The problem that is found next is that block encryption schemes are not vigorous to noise. The data integrity preservation is the third problem (Puech, Chaumont, & Strauss, 2008). The combination of encryption and watermarking can solve these types of problems.

Use of cryptography in images will make pixel intensity information to be transmitted in a form different from the original details so that only authorized personnel can view the image by using proper key and validate the image data. Thus image data included in as pixel information to be transmitted into an illegible form by different image encryption techniques as discussed above. Apart from these there are many more types of algorithms used for incorporating the image encryption. Different techniques of image encryption are incorporated that preserves the security of images. Algorithms based on both chaos and non-chaos image encryption schemes have been proposed. Of the both chaos based and non-chaos based, chaos is considered to be efficient and promising. The image encryption based on chaotic algorithm uses properties of dynamics that is deterministic and behavior that is not predictable. Encryption techniques are namely of three types permutation, reversal or replacement and techniques that include both substitution and transposition. There is change in the pixel values in substitution or replacement schemes while shuffling of pixel intensities is done in permutation. Improved security is uaranteed by combining both techniques. An image encryption scheme is proposed in (Guan, Huang, & Guan, 2005) which use Arnold cat map and Chen's chaotic system. Combinations of three permutation schemes is discussed, which can be in levels of bits, in levels of pixel and in block level permutations are introduced in any order (Mitra, Rao, & Prasanna, 2006). Key stream generator is added for enhancement in AES algorithm used in image encryption in (Zeghid et al., 2007). The scheme used in (Zhu, Z. L., Zhang, W., Wong, K. W., & Yu, H., 2011) does shuffling of bits which is chaos based. Shuffling of bits not only changes the position of bits of pixel intensities but also changes its pixel value. Total permutation is done in (Zhang, G., & Liu, Q., 2011) used for a novel encryption scheme for images. Security of encryption in images is improved by the combination of 2 logistic maps in (Ismail, Amin, & Diab, 2010). Multiple chaotic encryption systems are used in (Alsafasfeh & Arfoa, 2011). The custom image encryption schemes can be taken into account such as based on Rubik's cube and many more.

Digital Watermarking Approach

Watermarking is the process of embedding a signal into a multimedia content of text, image, audio or video types; and signal used as watermark can be of any format- text, image or audio signal. It can be viewed as a data hiding technique. The data hiding can be done in two domains - *spatial* and *frequency* domain. It can be basically reversible and irreversible. The properties to be satisfied by watermarking include robustness, capacity and imperceptibility. The robustness against attack is possible when the embedding is done in frequency domain and if capacity is of major concern spatial domain can be of great help. The message is imperceptibly embedded using watermarking and without any change in image size or format (Pal, Ghosh & Bhattacharya, 2013). In case of digital images, the information embedded can be either *invisible* or *visible* from the user perspective. As the security and confidentiality is primary concern, concentration is on imperceptible watermarks. Digital Watermarking technology is fit for being used as a form of copyright protection and a preventing those who have illegal in order intention to get a hold of confidential multimedia data including images disproportionately. The watermarking is based on spatial and frequency domain. *Reversible data hiding* focuses on data embedding and extraction (Zhang, X., 2011). There are number of schemes in spatial domain where additional data including images, notations are added within the encrypted image. In these schemes it's hopeful that original content is recovered without any change. In a scheme, watermarking is opted to share data (Coatrieux, G et al., 2000). When watermarking is applied to images, it allows the insertion of a message by modifying the pixel gray-scale values of the image in an imperceptible manner. Data-hiding is done in both steganography and watermarking with only a narrow line of difference in which watermarking safeguards the elimination of secret information in the cover medium whereas latter requires the existence of secret information to be unknown (Khan, A., Siddiqa, A., Munib, S., & Malik, S. A., 2014).

In the writing, a significant couple of calculations are anticipated to fulfill the property of changeableness. The ordinary techniques square measure upheld modulo 256 option used in (Puech, Chaumont & Strauss, 2008), lossless multi-determination revamp (Coatrieux, G., Le Guillou, C., Cauvin, J. M., & Roux, C., 2009), lossless pressure (Puech & Rodrigues, 2004), (Stinson, 2005), invertible commotion including (Schneier, 2007), qualification development (Cox et al., 1997), (William & Stallings, 2006),whole number undulating revamp (Coatrieux et al., 2000), alteration of histogram (Jaeger et al., 2014), then forward. All in all, these calculations target advanced pictures that square measure keeps as whole numbers from zero to 255. The best approach to reversibly floating so as to bring information into the items diagrammatically or settled point numbers, similar to the 3D models comprising of directions (e.g., (Zhang, X., 2011).) furthermore the high-dynamic-range pictures as indicated by (Acharya, R., Bhat, P. S., Kumar, S., & Min, L. C, 2003), has once in a while been explored. Be that as it may, reversible hiding in any style of learning is interesting to maintain a strategic distance from information misfortune. Since the vast majority of the overarching procedures trade out of the attributes of advanced pictures, straightforwardly floating so as to apply them to the articles diagrammatical or settled point numbers may experience troubles or cause an outsized contortion. In the preparatory work (Khan, A., Siddiqa, A., Munib, S., & Malik, S. A., 2014), the idea of keeping the balance information inside of the watermarked article is embraced in quantization-based inserting. Moreover, we tend to execute it on 3D network models so the main lattice model will pretty much be recouped. The condition for the exact recuperation is given in (Zhang, W., Ma, K., & Yu, N., 2014), furthermore the recuperation strategy might be performed with no particular information of the primary article. Indeed, even along these lines, it's capability to gauge the quantizer used inside of the regulation by the connected arithmetic investigation of the watermarked object, as appeared inside of the accompanying segment. Hence, the insurance of the algorithmic project must be expanded to thwart the potential data escape from the watermarked object.

Crypto-Watermarking Approaches

The method recognized in (Qian & Zhang, 2014) is one of the scheme of crypto-watermarking in which data hiding is done in encrypted images. The stream cipher technique for encryption followed by data hiding in which chosen bits are taken from the encoded picture to implant the mystery information.

Zhang, W., Ma, K., and Yu, N. (2014) had advised a scheme in which certain pixels are selected for estimating the errors and data hiding is done into these estimated errors. Standard stream cipher algorithm AES is used to encrypt the pixels of the image and special scheme is used to encrypt the estimation errors. The efficiency and feasibility of the scheme is computed by PSNR and embedding rate.

Pal, K., Ghosh, G., and Bhattacharya, M. (2013) had embedded the patient record including patient's name, diagnostic and region of interest into the cover image by the use of discrete cosine transform in frequency domain and RSA public-private key algorithm The infected region to be the ROI is detected through an amalgamation of contour detection algorithm and region growing. The embedded information is found to be obtained with exact similarity even from several attacked image.

The scheme described in Lakrissi, Y., Erritali, M., and Fakir, M. (2013) is based on the arrangement of encryption algorithms using secret keys and public-private keys including watermarking. The algorithm for image encryption is done using stream cipher technique with secret key encrypted with an asymmetric cipher technique. The watermarking algorithm is used to insert this encrypted secret key into the encrypted image.

The system explained by Bouslimi et al. (2012) moves towards a watermarking algorithm which is substitutive, the quantization index modulation (QIM) and an encryption algorithm which is stream or block cipher technique. In Joint Watermarking/Encryption scheme watermark is embedded during the encryption process. It allows verifying the image reliability in both encrypted and spatial domains. Here encryption and data embedding is conducted together at the stage for protection, decryption and data extraction can be applied in parallel.

The Medical image watermarking preserves image quality that is mandatory for medical diagnosis and treatment in Rao and Kumari (2011) highlights needs that are essential for medical image watermarking with a go over of developments since 2000 and simulated experiments to exhibit the significance of watermarking in management of medical information.

Puech, Chaumont, and Strauss (2008) portrayed the framework with encryption or information concealing calculations, the assurance of media information. The transmission time can be decreased by the utilization of the information pressure. This work, give answers for consolidate picture encryption and pressure. Utilization of reversible information concealing calculations on encoded pictures wish to evacuate the implanted data before the decoding of picture. The utilization of bit substitution-information concealing strategy helps for this reason. Keeping in mind the end goal to evacuate the watermarked information amid the unscrambling step, nearby standard deviation examination of the watermarked scrambled pictures is finished. Sharing of therapeutic picture in applications, for example, remote analysis help or e-learning, Coatrieux, g., Le Guillou, C., Cauvin, J. M., and Roux, C. (2009) proposes to make the picture more usable while watermarking it with related information digest. Watermarking is utilized to push in the Knowledge Digest (KD) into the dim scale pixel estimations of the related pictures. When it is shared through web, watermarking transmits dependability verifications of a picture and it's KD.

CRYPTO-WATERMARKING

Technologies are evolving for providing security to multimedia applications especially medical data or images that needs proper confidentiality, integrity and authenticity to be ensured. The popular among these technologies include combinations of cryptography and digital watermarking. Cryptographic methods and primitives allow access that is conditional for the protection of multimedia applications and data. The robustness of digital watermarking enables the data that is confidential cannot be removed or destroyed.

Challenges

Cryptography and watermarking are married in the system for crypto-watermarking (Sadeghi, 2008). To deal with various security issues in multimedia applications Crypto-Watermarking is one of the measures that involves great deal of study. The application which is in concern with current chapter work is health care imagery means. The major challenge posed by the system involves secure hiding of confidential information and proper extraction of the data in untrusted environment. The ownership proofs are also on the issues that must be dealt with these systems. The use of encryption and decryption using stream or block ciphers help in protection of data or images corresponding to the medical imagery. The chapter focuses on the works with combination of cryptographic and data hiding schemes so that it enables not to reveal sensitive data other than for those authorized to do so.

In application scenarios the watermark embedding phase requires the watermark extraction phase to know the key or the watermark itself for extraction of the information. This includes the dispute for ownership which can be relatively resolved by the use of public private crypto-system for encryption of secret key or watermark. Limitation in robustness of watermarking undermines the security.

Another challenge in this system is that the encryption and watermarking mechanisms should with stand compression. Because of this, medical mages cannot be communicated when this kind of risk persists. The solution to this kind of problem is encryption (Puech, 2008). Many techniques for encryption of images and data exist. In this chapter the need of the cryptographic and watermarking principles essential to confirm the security of medical imageries and statistics is discussed.

Applications

The application that makes use of Crypto-Watermarking System includes defense, health care institutions for medical imagery. The promise to the protection of medical images during transfer and during the archiving is the main objective. Watermarking accompanied by cryptography in medical imagery helps in increasing the security and provide authentication. Applications can vary from biomedicine, radiology, teradialogy in medicine and plenty more. Health data management can be done properly through multiple watermarking and secret key encryptions.

Case Study

The case study for this method systematically does the encryption and watermarking of medical images efficiently with confidentiality assured. A scheme for reversible crypto-watermarking for safe transfer of images include the biomedical image to be encrypted and the key used for encryption is subsequently ELGamal encrypted for confidentiality and security policy implication preservation. A medical image is selected for transmission in scenario of practioner and medical specialist. Before transmission following steps are done systematically. This constitutes encryption of image based on secret key using stream cipher method RC4. Then the encrypted image is watermarked using spread spectrum coding in DCT after the key itself being encrypted using public-private crypto-system. The encrypted and watermarked image is finally transmitted. The proposed methodology is depicted using a detailed diagram (*Figure 1*). Encrypting images using asymmetric methods are not suitable because they are computationally complex. So a conventional symmetric key encryption, with channel to transfer the key is used (Lakrissi, Y., Erritali, M., & Fakir, M., 2013). The projected method combines algorithm for symmetric image encryption, secret key encryption using asymmetric public-private scheme and spread spectrum coding algorithm in discrete cosine transform for watermarking. RSA being the traditional asymmetric method based on public-private keys and being probe to several security issues, the secret key is encrypted using ELGamal public-private cryptosystem.

Combining image or data encryption with watermarking technique for reliable transmission of medical images including scan and other medical informations and ensuring confidentiality and authenticity is the major intention to address.

- Encryption and Watermarking is the most combined techniques for safe transmission of images (Qian, Z., & Zhang, X., 2014).
- Efficient crypto-system is most essential for secure transmission.
- Stream cipher – symmetric key cipher is used due to it benefits for image encryption.

Figure 1. Proposed methodology

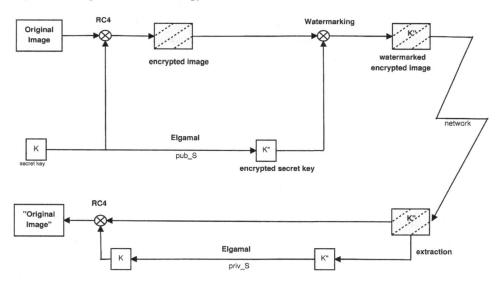

- ElGamal being stronger crypto-system due to randomization employed is more resistant to attacks and could be replaced for traditional RSA crypto-system used (Stinson, D. R., 2005).
- The quick analysis and extraction of medical images also requires confidentiality to be preserved.
- Because of the addition of noise by the any watermarking methodology, Robust Spread spectrum approach which reduces the noise input to images need to be employed

Basically, four steps are basically involved in the case study conducted for studying the crypto-watermarking technique. This is general methodology which could be revisited in various orders a further extension to this method is incorporated through the encryption of electronic patient record (EPR) into encrypted or non-encrypted images which can be done as part of future extension, a certain portion of this is carried out here. So general methodology is as follows:

1. Image encryption
2. Key encryption
3. Watermarking the encrypted key.
4. Transmission and reception of encrypted image.

1. Image Encryption

The utilization of internet for information transmissions has created the basic call for security. Several robust encryption techniques for plain messages have been developed to supply this demand. The encryption practice can be asymmetric, symmetric or hybrid. It can be functional to blocks or streams. The block encryption scheme applied to images, can meet with basically three inconveniences. The first and foremost one is when there is encryption of identical zones, they are found to be similar. The problem that is found next is that block encryption schemes are not vigorous to noise. The data integrity preservation is the third problem (Puech, Chaumont, & Strauss, 2008). The combination of encryption and watermarking can solve these types of difficulties. The brief idea of the encrypting method is elaborated in *Figure 2*. For X_i is considered to be poised of all N pixels of an image, RC4 encryption algorithm is applied. The encryption function is based on following equation shown in Equation 1. The encryption function can differ based on the algorithm used. The proposed work is done on RC4 algorithm and encryption of key is done on public-private key algorithm- ELGamal

$$Y = E_k(X)$$

Figure 2. Encryption and Watermarking

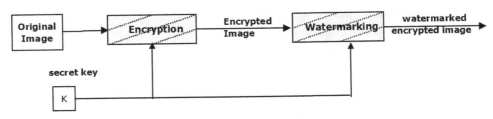

where $E_k()$ is the purpose for encryption with k as the secret key and Y is the equivalent cipher-text. The RC4 stream cipher method used is explained in following section especially the key generation and XOR operation.

a. Stream Cipher - RC4

RC4 could be a radial cipher designed for RSA Security in 1987 by West Chadic Rivest. It's a stream cipher algorithmic rule with variable key size, simple and very quick. Usually Stream cipher algorithms are accustomed to assemble the bits of plain text with a secret key stream of bits issued from a Pseudo Random Number Generator (PRNG), with typical use of XOR operation. The generation of key depends on one key which remains a secret, creating stream cipher algorithms as a part of varied techniques for radial coding. The specificity of such stream cipher algorithmic rule strictly depends on, however the bit key stream is created by the PRNG. The RC4 PRNG encompasses 2 steps:

1.   Initialization
2.   Byte key stream generation.

Key Scheduling Algorithm

To begin, the entries of S are set adequate to the values from zero through 255 in ascending order; that is; S[0] contains zero, S[1] contains 1 and so on. A variable T, which is a vector, is booted up. Now taking a key of length to be 256 bytes, which is transferred to variable T. Else if the length is different one, the first subsequent length of key is changed to components of T and then K is perennial as again and again so as to fill the vector T. These preliminary operations are briefed as in *Table 1.*

    After which a gentle swapping is done to get permuted result.

Byte Stream Generation

The input key is not used once Sb is given a initial permuted value. The generation of stream includes starting with Sb[0] and going up to to Sb[255], and, replacing

Table 1. Key scheduling step

```
for j = 0 to 255 do
Sb[j] = j;
Tb[j] = Key[j mod len];
```

Sb[i] with alternative byte takes place for all S[i] per a theme as configured of S. This process repeats as method continues.

This process generates a sequence of pseudo-random values. Then the input stream is XORed with the pseudo-random values produced by the algorithm. The encryption and decryption process is the same as the process of XORing data stream with the generated key sequence. If it is fed in an encrypted message, i decrypted message will be generated as output, and if it is fed in plain text message, it will produce the encrypted version (William & Stallings, 2006).

In RC4 module each value of k is generated based on RC4 key stream generation algorithm and the entries in S box are once again permuted. Encryption is done by XORing the key value k with the bytes of plain text image pixels. Decryption is done again by XORing the key value k cipher text rounding based on bytes.

2. Key Encryption

The secret key taken based on PRNG is the key to decrypt the medical image sent to the specialist so that he can view the image for diagnosis or further processing, so there is a great need to secure this key at the same time the key needs to be obtained by the specialist fast. The security is guaranteed through public-private key algorithm. In order to increase the security the proposed method use a strong algorithm known as ELGamal which increases the randomization involved in the cipher text also it is difficult against cryptanalysis. The practioner M takes the public key of Specialist S and encrypts the secret key and embeds the encrypted secret key in image using either watermarking or steganography principles. The basics of ELGamal crypto-system is explained in detail in following subsection.

a. ELGamal Cryptosystem

An ELGamal crypto-system functions in a very finite cyclic cluster group (Schneier, 1996) (Diffie & Hellman, 1976). An ELGamal cryptosystem are often represented by a 4-tuple (p, g, x, y), wherever p may be a massive prime and describes that group or cluster Z_p is employed, g is a part of order n in Z_p, x may be a random integer with $1<=x<=n-1$, and $y = g^x$. The steps within the ELGamal crypto-system area unit as follows:

1. Key generation: Pick a massive prime p, generator g of Z_p, private key is a random x such that $1<=x<=p-2$ and public key is 4 tuple (p, g, y = g^xmod p).
2. Encryption: Pick random k such that, $1<=k<=n-1$and encryption function is defined as

$$E(m) = (g^k \bmod p, \ my^k \bmod p) = (\gamma, \delta)$$

3. Decryption: Given cipher text (γ, δ) , compute $\delta\gamma^{-x}\bmod p$ and recover m such that:

$$m = \delta\gamma^{-x}\bmod p$$

3. Watermarking the Encrypted Key

Digital Watermarking technology is fit for being used as a form of copyright protection and a preventing those who have illegal in order intention to get a hold of confidential multimedia data including images disproportionately. The watermarking is based on spatial and frequency domain (Cox, Miller, Bloom, & Honsinger, 2002). The frequency domain being more robust to attacks, the work is done on Discrete Cosine Transform. The encrypted secret key is embedded in DCT domain using spread spectrum approach a traditional method discussed by (Cox, Kilian, Leighton & Shamoon, 1997) as the basic watermarking principle. For an input image, the DCT frequency components are computed using the Equation. 4 shown below:

$$y(u,v) = \sqrt{\frac{2}{M}}\sqrt{\frac{2}{N}}C_u C_v \sum\nolimits_{u=0}^{M-1}\sum\nolimits_{v=0}^{N-1} x(m,n)\cos\frac{(2m+1)u\pi}{2M}\cos\frac{(2n+1)u\pi}{2N}$$

In the equation, with size of N x M pixels, $x(m,n)$ is the spatial intensity at corresponding position of the image, and is the DCT frequency coefficient at corresponding point of the DCT matrix.

The inverse DCT operation is done for watermarked image to restore the image to cover image extracting the watermark information applying the Equation 5 shown below:

$$x(m,n) = \sqrt{\frac{2}{M}}\sqrt{\frac{2}{N}}C_u C_v \sum\nolimits_{u=0}^{M-1}\sum\nolimits_{v=0}^{N-1} y(u,v)\cos\frac{(2m+1)u\pi}{2M}\cos\frac{(2n+1)u\pi}{2N}$$

Vital visual details are included in low frequency bands of the image and geometrical modifications could eliminate high frequency coefficients of the image – basically compression. The watermark is embedded by changing the frequency elements of the mid –band frequencies so that the visual excellence of the image will not be distorted and the watermark cannot be removed by geometrical changes.

a. Spread Spectrum Watermarking

The proposed watermarking calculation in the change area i.e. DCT space is spread range system. In the first place, the best place for supplement the watermark bits is found by file sorting for getting the primary n high recurrence coefficients. The watermark is spread over to numerous containers gathering recurrence so that the vitality in any canister is insignificant and can't be recognized. The watermark ought not be set in locales of inconsequentiality. Watermark is known as a sign transmitted through the recurrence space of the picture. The vigor and security of watermark is guaranteed by, setting the watermark expressly in the most noteworthy coefficients of the picture perceptually. Keeping in mind the end goal to place watermark of length n into a NxN picture, coefficients are registered for the NxN picture utilizing DCT and setting the watermark into extent coefficients with high values. Make a watermark where every worth xi is picked freely as per N (0, 1). The extricated from host advanced picture, an arrangement of qualities Vi, into which a watermark xi is embedded to acquire a balanced grouping of qualities Wi. Watermark insertion results in watermarked image W, with a scaling parameter α used to specify, the extent to which watermark alters the cover image. Formula for computing watermarked signal is shown in Equation 6. A large value of α will cause perceptual degradation in the watermarked image.

$$W_i = V_i = \alpha x_i$$

where V_i is DCT coefficient value of the image and α is scaling factor denotes the imperceptibility degree. The extraction is reverse of the process of insertion including deviation analysis. For each watermarked cipher text Y_i, applying the decoding function for two possible values (0 or 1) while analyzing the local standard deviation. The bit value is selected where local standard deviation is least.

4. Transmission and Reception of Encrypted Image

Transmission and reception includes the last phase of the Crypto-Watermarking system when the sender transmits the medical image with secret data watermarked which can be secret key or any other patient record whose confidentiality and integrity needs to be assured. The intended recipient actually extracts the watermark which includes the confidential data as well as the key to decrypt it. After which he or she could view the imagery.

SOLUTIONS AND RECOMMENDATIONS

The reversible crypto-watermarking system has been implemented using python - OpenCV library running on an Ubuntu 14.04 platform with the support of Intel core 3 and 4GB RAM. The performance of each step in combined crypto-watermarking techniques is evaluated using the dataset described in next section.

1. Dataset

The reversible crypto-watermarking approach is applied on more than 200 gray level images that are obtained from one (Candemir et al., 2014) (Jaeger et al., 2014) and other sources. The proposed method is applied on a chest image (396 x 400 pixels) and the medical image (512 x 512 pixels) which is shown in Figure 3 and in Figure 4 respectively. The watermark data is encrypted key data which is variable length ranging up to 126bits. The results are evaluated using mean-square-error (MSE), peak-signal-to noise- ratio (PSNR) and entropy for evaluating encryption efficiency.

Figure 3. First input

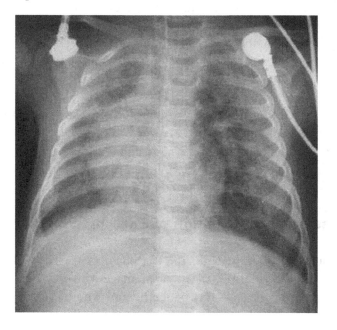

Figure 4. Second input

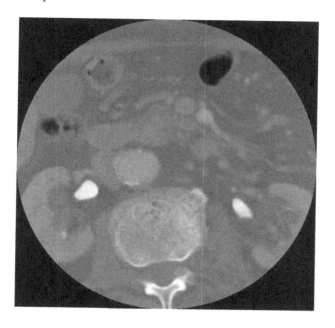

2. Comparison and Evaluation

Stream cipher method is applied to encrypt the input image. The encryption of the original image Figure 3 is done by using the RC4 algorithm to get the encrypted image illustrated in *Figure 5*. Using stream cipher method shows just few seconds as time for encryption. In this encrypted image, bits of encrypted key are embedded to get the watermarked encrypted image illustrated in *Figure 6*. On reception of image by the specialist the watermark is extracted from the image which is embedded secret key k' and this secret key is used to decrypt the image to view the initial image. The watermark extracted image and corresponding decrypted image is shown in *Figure 7* and *Figure 8* respectively.

The *Table 2* shows the execution time for each step done on input images *Figure 3* and *Figure 4*.

3. Results

In order to interpret the results obtained, it is necessary to develop tools to measure the error between embedded and original image. Among these strategies histogram analysis, entropy analysis and PSNR ratios respectively are used. Gray image is having 256 gray scale levels and the theoretical value of entropy is 8bits. Entropy is

Figure 5. Encrypted image

Figure 6. Watermarked image

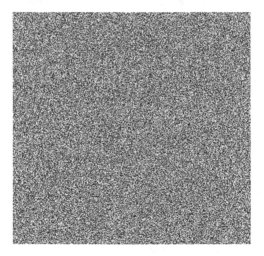

issue to know the security and strength concerned within the cryptography method for images. Entropy for encrypted image is near 7.9bits/pixel. *Table 3* shows the entropy of input image and encrypted image respectively.

A histogram is a graphical representation of a continuous variable distribution. So the difference can be noted clearly from the histogram of original images and encrypted image shown in *Figure 9* and *Figure 10* respectively. Uniform distribution of pixels are done, which can resist attacks. So, efficiency of algorithm is ensured

Figure 7. Key Extracted image

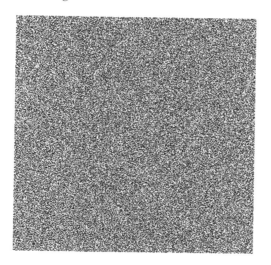

Figure 8. Decrypted image

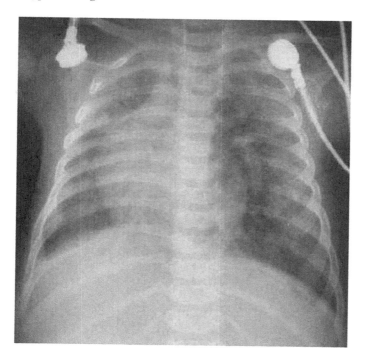

Table 2. *Execution time for rc4*

RC4 – Image Encrytion	First Image	Second Image
Time	3 msec	2.3msec

Table 3. *Entropy for medical image and its encrypted image*

Image	Entropy(bits/pixel)
Chest image	7.21
Encrypted image	7.99

due to the security it guarantees with secure transmission of confidential information.

By the comparison of both histograms that of the initial image, Figure 9 and that of the image encrypted, Figure 10, with remark that the probabilities of occurrence of gray levels in the image are equally distributed also shown respectively.

4. Quality Analysis

The proposed crypto-watermarking system is applied to chest image. Quality Metrics used is Peak Signal to Noise Ratio and to evaluate the similarity between the

Figure 9. *Histogram(chest)*

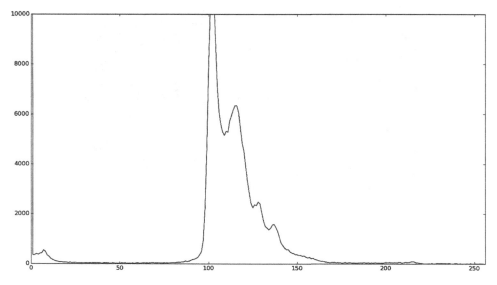

Figure 10. Histogram(Encrypted)

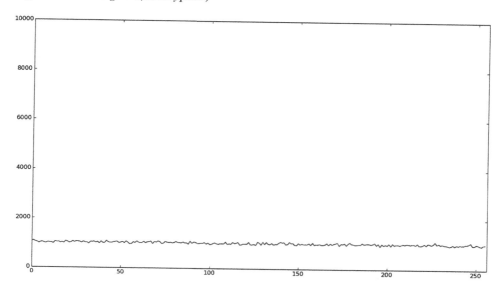

Decrypted image and original image. Bigger is PSNR, better is quality of image. PSNR for image with size M x N is given by Equation 7:

$$PSNR = 10\log_{10}\left(\frac{\sum\limits_{x=1}^{M}\sum\limits_{y=1}^{N}E^2_{max}}{\sum\limits_{x=1}^{M}\sum\limits_{y=1}^{N}(f(x,y)-f'(x,y))^2}\right)$$

where, $f(x,y)$ are pixel gray values of original image. $f'(x,y)$ is pixel gray values of watermarked image. M and N are image pixel dimensions. PSNR value obtained for the decrypted image is high.

The value for α is taken to be 0.5 in the whole experiment. For different values, the result is not accurate. The watermarked chest image shown in the *Figure: 6* shows a PSNR value of 70.18dB which is high compared to other approaches discussed in literature. If the amount of data embedded is increased to 15242 bits the same image shows a PSNR value of 61.08dB which is good value with less distortion in image quality. Decryption of key involves the authentication through the ELGamal crypto-system thereby safeguarding the confidentiality in its reality.

INFERENCE

The combination of cryptography, information-hiding and integrity verification is projected and evaluated for safe transmission of medical data with the individual image. The stream cipher technique is strong to moderate noise with top quality issue. Within the field of cryptography and image watermarking, crypto-watermarking is a vital space of analysis in medical mental imagery that helps in protecting confidentiality, genuineness and integrity of medical information. DCT domain is employed to embed the key attributable to its physical property and hardiness to geometric distortions. The management of magnitude relation between the capacity and distortion got to be addressed more that is initiated with our future analysis direction. The management of ratio between the capacity and distortion need to be addressed further which is initiated with our future research direction.

FUTURE RESEARCH DIRECTIONS

The following are some suggestions for future study.

- A comparative study between all the different Crypto-Watermarking schemes based on different encryption and data hiding schemes can be done.
- Proposed system can also be applied to other domains other than discrete cosine transform i.e. in prediction error domain of spatial system.
- Variety of techniques can be applied to eliminate the addition of unnecessary noise.

FUTURE CASE STUDY: EPR EMBEDDING IN SPATIAL DOMAIN

In EPR embedding, the EPR encrypted data is embedded into the cover image based on prediction errors exploiting the sorting according to the local variances μ. The local variance $\mu_{i,j}$ has several features like this value remain unchanged after data hiding also this value is proportional to the magnitude of prediction error of the cell under consideration. Cell is unit of pixels in which data should be embedded. Using the prediction scheme allows efficient embedding of data with low distortion. Each pixel of the cover image can be used for data hiding, so capacity can be increased considerably. Low prediction error values are ideal for data hiding.

The security priorities have increased with increased use of computer networks and wireless technologies. EPR data include various patient information that is relevant for the medical treatment, through its communication can be used for proper diagnostics by opinion gathering. Data include notes from physicians, scan reports - MRIs, CT scan, and clinical observation results. The patient's data can be accessed by medical specialist, by the patient at home, and other medical practitioners. This can help improve overall quality of health care delivery; the welfares of this technology must be well-adjusted with the privacy and security implications. Thus encryption, access control mechanisms are used to safeguard the EPR data for facilitating. Techniques of message encryption have been developed to meet this demand. The original image is embedded with EPR data encrypted using a secret key. This encrypted data is embedded with cover image and transferred to the network. The transferred image is received and the encrypted data is extracted reversibly before which the hash is calculated and compared with the extracted hash value. The integrity check is done here. Also the algorithm must be lossless scheme for extracting the encrypted data properly. With the secret key decryption of EPR data is done.

CONCLUSION

In the field of cryptography and image watermarking, crypto-watermarking is an important area of research in medical imagery which helps in preserving security, confidentiality, authenticity and integrity of medical data. It's a process of enabling data hiding by the aid of encryption. Encryption is done using various methods which can be block cipher or stream cipher. Watermarking of the encrypted data or image can be done in various domains taking into account various features of respective domain and it depends on the applications that perform.

The proposed Crypto-Watermarking System processed the medical images for its safe transfer. Encryption of image using standard stream cipher algorithm is done which is very fast and reliable. Being robust to moderate noise stream cipher algorithm is efficient with high quality factor. The secret key used for encryption is then watermarked in DCT domain by the use of spread spectrum coding algorithm due to its imperceptibility and robustness to geometric distortions. The additional security is guaranteed by the use of ELGamal public-private key crypto-system for secret key encryption which is stronger than traditional RSA system. The system is verified using 250 input images and result is presented and high PSNR value obtained concludes the method to be efficient. Future work is to try the same on various other transform domains and by increasing the embedding rate.

REFERENCES

Acharya, R., Bhat, P. S., Kumar, S., & Min, L. C. (2003). Transmission and storage of medical images with patient information. *Computers in Biology and Medicine*, *33*(4), 303–310. doi:10.1016/S0010-4825(02)00083-5 PMID:12791403

Alsafasfeh, Q. H., & Arfoa, A. A. (2011). Image encryption based on the general approach for multiple chaotic systems. *Journal of Signal and Information Processing*, *2*(03), 238–244. doi:10.4236/jsip.2011.23033

Bouslimi, D., Coatrieux, G., Cozic, M., & Roux, C. (2012). A joint encryption/watermarking system for verifying the reliability of medical images. *Information Technology in Biomedicine. IEEE Transactions on*, *16*(5), 891–899.

Candemir, S., Jaeger, S., Palaniappan, K., Musco, J. P., Singh, R. K., Xue, Z., & McDonald, C. J. et al. (2014). Lung segmentation in chest radiographs using anatomical atlases with nonrigid registration. *IEEE Transactions on Medical Imaging*, *33*(2), 577–590. doi:10.1109/TMI.2013.2290491 PMID:24239990

Celik, M. U., Sharma, G., & Saber, E. (2002). Reversible data hiding. In *Image Processing. 2002. Proceedings. 2002 International Conference on* (Vol. 2, pp. II-157). IEEE. doi:10.1109/ICIP.2002.1039911

Cheung, Y. M., & Wu, H. T. (2007). A sequential quantization strategy for data embedding and integrity verification. *Circuits and Systems for Video Technology. IEEE Transactions on*, *17*(8), 1007–1016.

Coatrieux, G., Le Guillou, C., Cauvin, J. M., & Roux, C. (2009). Reversible watermarking for knowledge digest embedding and reliability control in medical images. *Information Technology in Biomedicine. IEEE Transactions on*, *13*(2), 158–165.

Coatrieux, G., Maitre, H., Sankur, B., Rolland, Y., & Collorec, R. (2000). Relevance of watermarking in medical imaging. In *Information Technology Applications in Biomedicine, 2000. Proceedings. 2000 IEEE EMBS International Conference on* (pp. 250-255). IEEE. doi:10.1109/ITAB.2000.892396

Cox, I., Miller, M., Bloom, J., Fridrich, J., & Kalker, T. (2007). *Digital watermarking and steganography*. Morgan Kaufmann.

Cox, I. J., Kilian, J., Leighton, F. T., & Shamoon, T. (1997). Secure spread spectrum watermarking for multimedia. *Image Processing. IEEE Transactions on*, *6*(12), 1673–1687.

Cox, I. J., Miller, M. L., Bloom, J. A., & Honsinger, C. (2002). *Digital watermarking* (Vol. 53). San Francisco: Morgan Kaufmann.

De Vleeschouwer, C., & Macq, B. (2003). Circular interpretation of bijective transformations in lossless watermarking for media asset management. *Multimedia. IEEE Transactions on*, 5(1), 97–105.

Diffie, W., & Hellman, M. E. (1976). New directions in cryptography. *Information Theory. IEEE Transactions on*, 22(6), 644–654.

Fernández-Alemán, J. L., Señor, I. C., Lozoya, P. Á. O., & Toval, A. (2013). Security and privacy in electronic health records: A systematic literature review. *Journal of Biomedical Informatics*, 46(3), 541–562. doi:10.1016/j.jbi.2012.12.003 PMID:23305810

Fridrich, J., Goljan, M., & Du, R. (2001, August). Invertible authentication. In Photonics West 2001-Electronic Imaging (pp. 197-208). International Society for Optics and Photonics.

Goljan, M., Fridrich, J. J., & Du, R. (2001, January). Distortion-free data embedding for images. In *Information Hiding* (pp. 27–41). Springer Berlin Heidelberg. doi:10.1007/3-540-45496-9_3

Guan, Z. H., Huang, F., & Guan, W. (2005). Chaos-based image encryption algorithm. *Physics Letters. [Part A]*, 346(1), 153–157. doi:10.1016/j.physleta.2005.08.006

Honsinger, C. W., Jones, P. W., Rabbani, M., & Stoffel, J. C. (2001). *U.S. Patent No. 6,278,791*. Washington, DC: U.S. Patent and Trademark Office.

Ismail, I. A., Amin, M., & Diab, H. (2010). A digital image encryption algorithm based a composition of two chaotic logistic maps. *International Journal of Network Security*, 11(1), 1–10.

Jaeger, S., Karargyris, A., Candemir, S., Folio, L., Siegelman, J., Callaghan, F., & Thoma, G. et al. (2014). Automatic tuberculosis screening using chest radiographs. *IEEE Transactions on Medical Imaging*, 33(2), 233–245. doi:10.1109/TMI.2013.2284099 PMID:24108713

Khan, A., Siddiqa, A., Munib, S., & Malik, S. A. (2014). A recent survey of reversible watermarking techniques. *Information Sciences*, 279, 251–272. doi:10.1016/j.ins.2014.03.118

Lakrissi, Y., Erritali, M., & Fakir, M. (2013). A Joint Encryption/Watermarking Algorithm for Secure Image Transfer. *International Journal of Computer Networking and Communication*, 1(1). doi:10.1109/TCSVT.2015.2418611

Levoy, M., Pulli, K., Curless, B., Rusinkiewicz, S., Koller, D., Pereira, L., & Fulk, D. et al. (2000, July). The digital Michelangelo project: 3D scanning of large statues. In *Proceedings of the 27th annual conference on Computer graphics and interactive techniques* (pp. 131-144). ACM Press/Addison-Wesley Publishing Co. doi:10.1145/344779.344849

Macq, B., & Dewey, F. (1999, October). Trusted headers for medical images. In DFG VIII-D II Watermarking Workshop (Vol. 10). Erlangen.

Menezes, A. J., Van Oorschot, P. C., & Vanstone, S. A. (1996). *Handbook of applied cryptography*. CRC Press. doi:10.1201/9781439821916

Mitra, A., Rao, Y. S., & Prasanna, S. R. M. (2006). A new image encryption approach using combinational permutation techniques. *International Journal of Computer Science*, *1*(2), 127–131.

Ni, Z., Shi, Y. Q., Ansari, N., & Su, W. (2006). Reversible data hiding. *Circuits and Systems for Video Technology. IEEE Transactions on*, *16*(3), 354–362.

Pal, K., Ghosh, G., & Bhattacharya, M. (2013, December). A new combined crypto-watermarking technique using RSA algorithm and discrete cosine transform to retrieve embedded EPR from noisy bio-medical images. In *Condition Assessment Techniques in Electrical Systems (CATCON), 2013 IEEE 1st International Conference on* (pp. 368-373). IEEE.

Pérez-Freire, L., Comesana, P., & Pérez-González, F. (2005, January). Information-theoretic analysis of security in side-informed data hiding. In *Information Hiding* (pp. 131–145). Springer Berlin Heidelberg. doi:10.1007/11558859_11

Pérez-Freire, L., & Pérez-González, F. (2009). Spread-spectrum watermarking security. *Information Forensics and Security. IEEE Transactions on*, *4*(1), 2–24.

Puech, W. (2008, October). An Efficient Hybrid Method for Safe Transfer of Medical Images. In E-MEDISYS'08: E-Medical Systems.

Puech, W., Chaumont, M., & Strauss, O. (2008, February). A reversible data hiding method for encrypted images. In *Electronic Imaging 2008* (pp. 68191E–68191E). International Society for Optics and Photonics.

Puech, W., & Rodrigues, J. M. (2004, September). A new crypto-watermarking method for medical images safe transfer. In *Signal Processing Conference, 2004 12th European* (pp. 1481-1484). IEEE.

Qian, Z., & Zhang, X. (2014). *Reversible Data Hiding in Encrypted Image with Distributed Source Encoding*. Academic Press.

Rao, N. V., & Kumari, V. M. (2011). Watermarking in medical imaging for security and authentication. *Information Security Journal: A Global Perspective, 20*(3), 148-155.

Sadeghi, A. R. (2008). The marriage of cryptography and watermarking—beneficial and challenging for secure watermarking and detection. In *Digital Watermarking* (pp. 2–18). Springer Berlin Heidelberg. doi:10.1007/978-3-540-92238-4_2

Schneier, B. (1996). *Applied cryptography.* New York: Wiley.

Schneier, B. (2007). *Applied cryptography: protocols, algorithms, and source code in C.* John Wiley & Sons.

Shahid, Z., Chaumont, M., & Puech, W. (2011). Fast protection of H. 264/AVC by selective encryption of CAVLC and CABAC for I and P frames. *Circuits and Systems for Video Technology. IEEE Transactions on, 21*(5), 565–576.

Stinson, D. R. (2005). *Cryptography: theory and practice.* CRC Press.

Thodi, D. M., & Rodriguez, J. J. (2004, October). Prediction-error based reversible watermarking. In *Image Processing, 2004. ICIP'04. 2004 International Conference on* (Vol. 3, pp. 1549-1552). IEEE. doi:10.1109/ICIP.2004.1421361

Tian, J. (2003). Reversible data embedding using a difference expansion. *IEEE Transactions on Circuits and Systems for Video Technology, 13*(8), 890–896. doi:10.1109/TCSVT.2003.815962

William, S., & Stallings, W. (2006). *Cryptography and Network Security, 4/E.* Pearson Education India.

Wu, H. T., & Cheung, Y. M. (2005, September). A reversible data hiding approach to mesh authentication. In *Web Intelligence, 2005. Proceedings. The 2005 IEEE/WIC/ACM International Conference on* (pp. 774-777). IEEE.

Wu, H. T., & Cheung, Y. M. (2010). Reversible watermarking by modulation and security enhancement. *Instrumentation and Measurement. IEEE Transactions on, 59*(1), 221–228.

Xuan, G., Zhu, J., Chen, J., Shi, Y. Q., Ni, Z., & Su, W. (2002). Distortionless data hiding based on integer wavelet transform. *Electronics Letters, 38*(25), 1646–1648. doi:10.1049/el:20021131

Zeghid, M., Machhout, M., Khriji, L., Baganne, A., & Tourki, R. (2007). A modified AES based algorithm for image encryption. *International Journal on Computer Science and Engineering, 1*(1), 70–75.

Zhang, G., & Liu, Q. (2011). A novel image encryption method based on total shuffling scheme. *Optics Communications*, *284*(12), 2775–2780. doi:10.1016/j.optcom.2011.02.039

Zhang, W., Ma, K., & Yu, N. (2014). Reversibility improved data hiding in encrypted images. *Signal Processing*, *94*, 118–127. doi:10.1016/j.sigpro.2013.06.023

Zhang, X. (2011). Reversible data hiding in encrypted image. *Signal Processing Letters, IEEE*, *18*(4), 255–258. doi:10.1109/LSP.2011.2114651

Zhu, Z. L., Zhang, W., Wong, K. W., & Yu, H. (2011). A chaos-based symmetric image encryption scheme using a bit-level permutation. *Information Sciences*, *181*(6), 1171–1186. doi:10.1016/j.ins.2010.11.009

KEY TERMS AND DEFINITIONS

Computer Vision: It is an area that contains procedures for obtaining, handling, examining, and understanding images and, high dimensional facts from the real world in order to produce mathematical or representational data.

Crypto-Watermarking: Crypto-Watermarking is the synonym used for techniques which binds watermarking with cryptographic features.

Digital Watermarking: Digital watermarking is a convenient way of embedding covertly noises into multimedia signals such as an audio, video or image data. It is typically used to identify ownership of the copyright of such signal.

Discrete Cosine Transform: The discrete cosine transform (DCT) is a technique for converting a signal into elementary frequency components. It is widely used in image compression. Here we develop some simple functions to compute the DCT and to compress images.

Encryption: It is an effective method for data security in which one converts the data into a form that is not easily understood called the cipher text. Data encrypted can be accessed by secret key or passwords that allows subsequent decryption of encrypted file. File that is not encrypted is called plain text.

Health Insurance Portability and Accountability Act (HIPAA): Efficiency and effectiveness of health care system was ensured by the act enacted by United States Congress on August 21 1996.

Peak-Signal-to-Noise-Ratio(PSNR): The term peak signal-to-noise ratio (PSNR) is an expression for the ratio between the maximum possible value (power) of a signal and the power of distorting noise that affects the quality of its representation.

Pseudo Random Number Generator (PRNG): Pseudo Random Number Generator is a random generator used to generate bits randomly that have properties similar to random numbers.

Steganography: Steganography is concerned with hiding secret data into the media.

Stream Cipher: A stream cipher is a symmetric key cipher where plaintext digits are combined with a pseudorandom cipher digit stream (key stream). In a stream cipher each plaintext digit is encrypted one at a time with the corresponding digit of the key stream, to give a digit of the cipher text stream.

Chapter 11

Personalized Neuro–Fuzzy Expert System for Determination of Nutrient Requirements

Priti Srinivas Sajja
Sardar Patel University, India

Jeegar Ashokkumar Trivedi
Sardar Patel University, India

ABSTRACT

In the modern fast and stressful life, an individual does not have time to take an extra care for one's self. Support from general information about health and nutrient requirement through modern computing infrastructure is very limited and common. Generic information on the Web and other media sometime raises genuine queries about the good health. Further, typical solutions available may not interact with users in friendly way and deal with vague inputs provided by users. To resolve this issue, a system is required which knows its users, acts smartly and friendly, learns from past data & history and provides customised advisory. This chapter introduces a neuro-fuzzy architecture, based on which an expert system for determination of nutrient requirements is presented. The chapter includes in depth literature survey, concepts, implementation details with sample code, neural network structure, fuzzy membership functions used, sample input–output screens of the system and future work.

DOI: 10.4018/978-1-5225-1002-4.ch011

INTRODUCTION

Traditionally happiness is defined as good health; and everybody wants to be happy! In the modern fast and stressful life, an individual may not have time to take an extra care for one's self. It is necessary to observe daily routine of a person and set nutrition need accordingly, which requires an expert's advice which many cannot afford. Though, everybody gets lot of information from the platform life Internet and the Web, such information is not much useful because every individual is different. Each needs a customised advice to plan one's health and set nutrition requirement accordingly without taking much trouble.

The advances of information and communication technology (ICT) can make this possible. The ICT enables use of various devices such as computers, mobiles and other machines with necessary supporting architecture such as networking, protocols, techniques, architectures and standards.

Many solutions exist to guide an individual for his routine healthcare since a long time. Most of them try to provide generalised information collected from various resources, stored at a given location in a very structured, predefined form and can be accessed in restricted manner. Commonly observed limitations of such systems can be given as follows.

- One has to collect, organise and store information at a given location in a rigid format;
- The information collected is common for everybody, hence only generalised solution can be offered by such system;
- Most of the systems are legacy and available on a single computer or a single device at doctor's clinic or expert's office;
- Most of the systems are mainly database oriented in nature and do not offer advantages of knowledge orientation; and
- Such systems do not take advantages of modern architecture such as cloud and grid.

There are some exceptions to the aforementioned observations. People have successfully implemented and used rule base expert systems on the Web. Such systems take advantage of latest infrastructural facilities such as the Web and also offer advantages related to added intelligence using expert system techniques. However, decision making about the personal need requires much more. It is difficult to generalise decision making process and hence requirements of users. It can be learn from the part experience and data. Further, user's inputs and experience data are vague in nature. This leads to utilization of a modern artificial intelligence techniques such as neural network and fuzzy logic in a hybrid fashion. Neuro-fuzzy hybridising can offer an impressive solution here. Considering this, following objectives can be set.

- There should be an architecture facilitating use of a hybrid neuro-fuzzy system for decision making. Such architecture may be used for other applications also in related domains;
- The architecture should operate on the Web, preferable cloud or closed knowledge grid, so that data and input from various distributed resources can be used in effective manner;
- A system is to be developed based on the architecture designed in such a way that it understands its users, learns from their behaviour and provides tailor made advisory to the users;
- The system should document user's information, data and knowledge about the business in a suitable ontology or structure;
- The system also should be capable of dealing with partial and fuzzy information as well as system should learn from the past data of users;
- Alternatively, such system may be operational on personal devises such as mobile and wearable computers.

To meet these objectives, the chapter proposes a neuro-fuzzy expert system for determination of nutrient requirements for one's health living in a very much personalised manner. The chapter documents information related to the proposed work in following way.

Section 1 of the chapter introduces the topic and establishes need of the proposed work by demonstrating the current scenario in brief. This section also presents a brief summary on the work documented in the chapter. Section 2 describes in depth literature survey and work done in the area at national and international level with common observations and limitations. Section 3 presents a brief discussion of the techniques and fundamentals used, which includes brief overview of fuzzy logic, artificial neural network and neuro-fuzzy hybridization in different way. Section 4 presents a broad architecture of the neuro-fuzzy expert system for decision making. An experiment, some sample codes, technical information related to implementation and input as well as output design of the system along with a few test cases are presented in section 5. Section 6 discusses the results and concludes with application of the research work in other areas, benefits and extension possible for future research work.

BRIEF SUMMARY OF THE WORK DONE

Mass nutrition requirement is common for human beings and uses popular mass media such as newspaper columns, magazine articles and general websites. However, as stated earlier, such general purpose information may not be useful for a particular user or group of users. Further, it requires more customised approach and special (more personalised) technology too. Automatic and nutrition requirement generally employed with tools such as computerised systems, mobile based systems and other such technologies which is more personalised and handy to the users. Many such systems are employed and experimented by various researchers at national and international level. Prominent of them are listed below.

Feskanich D, Sielaff BH, Chong K and Buzzard IM (1989) presented computerized collection and analysis of dietary intake information using a hierarchically arranged food descriptions within a simple database. The food items are encoded according to their ingredients, nutritious values and usage. Binary trees and physical pointers are employed in the system for efficient data retrieval. The system also uses real time interaction to make the system more effective (Feskanich, Sielaff, Chong, & Buzzard, 1989). At the same time, Levine JA, Madden AM, Morgan MY (1987) proposed validation of a computer based system for assessing dietary intake. They have used patients' dietary history from a few hospitals and developed a computerised system for collection of patient's data. They have extracted information from various experts to generate standard food tables to calculate the composition of nutrients. Immediately after a year, in 1989 a system for interpretation of dietary intake was proposed by Guthrie HA (1989). There were many more researchers who contributed in the field during this decade namely Frank GC (1985), Engle A, Lynn LL, Koury K and Boyar AP (1990) and Fong AK & Kretsch MJ (1990).

During the next decade, Sandström B (2001) developed a framework for food based dilatory system. This framework is designed for the European Union, which identifies major food resources for the nutrition required, suggests food patterns suitable with desirable nutrient intakes, and other guidelines such as frequency of intake, portion size, etc. Gould SM and Anderson J (2000) have used interactive multimedia system to disseminate nutrition education towards a special group of low income humans. Bakker I et al. (2003) presented some comments on computerization of a dietary history in their study. Future directions and current nutritional requirements are analysed by Dwyer J, Picciano MF and Raiten DJ (2003). They have considered the United States of America as their region for study. Yasmine Probst and Linda Tapsell (2005) did a full state of the art survey. Approximately 29 dietary assessment programs are presented with their brief description and evaluation.

Some latest systems are also available for individual use, for example, Nutrabalance (2014) provides a computerised nutritional analysis report for an individual.

One of its main focuses is on the analysis of the pathological laboratory findings and presenting them graphically for comparison. These results are later on used to custom design dietary requirements for an individual. Bueche J et al. (2008) has elaborated nutrition care process in detail and designed a model for the same. Hoggle LB et al. (2006) highlighted use of electronic media in nutritional analysis and advisory system. In a similar fashion, a dietetics practice framework is also designed and presented in the work of Julie O'Sullivan Maillet, Janet Skates and Ellen Pritchett (2005).

Sometimes counseling is also required with the users to help them understand the complicated numbers presented as nutritional standards. Such counseling helps an average person in understanding and practically applying the nutrition information they are provided. The method and result of the research work are documented in the work of Stein Karen (2010).

Ali Fahmi, Amin Dorostanian, Hassan Rezazadeh and Alireza Ostadrahimi (2013) developed an intelligent decision support system for nutrition therapy. They have designed an expert system for decision support in nutritional planning using rules in the systems knowledge base. These rules support fuzziness and approximate reasoning with help of fuzzy logic utility. Further, the system is integrated with artificial neural network for knowledge management to generate novel rules.

Besides the above listed solutions, there are so many domain specific systems which help in nutritional analysis and advisory. For specific disease such as diabetes, cancer, and kidney patients; for human beings with malnutrition effects, physically challenged users and special group of users such as pregnant women, etc; many solutions are available. Some common observation of the study can be listed as follows.

The system works on rigid and specific input and user interface is not much friendly. An average human being may not be aware of nutritional standards and units of the values. Further, he may be poor in describing the exact characteristics as well symptoms to the system.

Such system may not be capable of self-learning from the user's logs. Depending on user's response, the system should self-update the nutritional requirements, food portion and frequency of food intake. The general standards may not be appropriate to every individual. From the user's interaction, the system may set customised standards to the specific user and suggest advises.

The system should be designed in a manner that it can encash advantages of object oriented technology and platform independence. Further, in current era, majority has access to facility of the Internet (as well as World Wide Web, also called the Web) and mobile phones; such system should work on personalised devices such as mobile phones.

UNDERLYING TECHNOLOGIES

To design the proposed system, there is a need to employ latest technology such as fuzzy logic, neural network and neuro-fuzzy hybridization. Before the generic architecture is presented it is trivial for readers to understand the underlying concepts, which are described in this section.

Fuzzy Logic

If somebody asks you, 'Are you young?' what would you say? Most of us say yes, why not! However, the strength and confidence on the statement decreases as your age marches towards 100 years! One can not draw a rigid boundary and fix that if age of a person is 25 or less, then the person is young, otherwise not! In other words, a formal statement can be made that if age of a person is less than or equal to 25 years, then the person belongs to the class of young people. Mathematically the statement is written as follows:

Young = {(set of all) x, where Age(x) <=25 Years}

Here Young is the name of the set, which is a collection of persons denoted by x whose age is not more than or equal to 25 years. From the above definition, it is clear that if a person's age is 24 years then he is clearly and completely a member of the set. If age of a person is 25 years and just a single day, then certainly he is not a member of the set. That is, either a person is a member of the set or not is identified as 1 and 0 respectively. Such set is known as crisp set of binary set, as it gives true/false, yes/no, 1/0 or White/Black results only. Such a set can be a finite set, an infinite set or an empty set. Some examples are listed as follows:

- **Finite Set Example:** Set of all non-negative integers less than six. Clearly, the set contains 0, 1, 2, 3, 4, and 5 (remember 6 is not less than 6).
- **Infinite Set Example:** Set of all integers less than 6. There are many numbers which are less than 6. The numbers start with 5, 4, 3, 2, 1, 0, -1, -2, and so on. However, it is possible to determine if a number is member of a set of not.
- **Empty Sets:** Set of live fishes on earth. Obviously, the set has no members, hence the set is known as an empty set.

In reality, decision making and problem solving processes are not such rigid but vague and fuzzy. Belongingness to the set is not exactly either-or type of relationship. Lofty A Zadeh (1965) presented an ideal of partial belongingness to the set with the notion of fuzzy sets. Consider the example stated above illustrating set of young people. A two-year-old child is clearly a member of the set and ninety-year-old person is completely not a member of the set. What about 35 years 'young' lady? She would always prefer to be 'Young'. Another such example is warm water setting for a bathroom shower. The definition of warm is different from person to person in different regions and situations. According to the theory of Lofty A. Zadeh, such membership can be graded and gradual instead of complete and abrupt. This describes a fuzzy set. An individual items' grade is now not only 1 (completely belongs to the set) or 0 (does not belong to the set), but partially belongs to the set, which is denoted by a number between 1 and 0. This number is known as membership degree and generally denoted by the Greek letter μ. As the number increases, the membership degree to the set also increases. Now the fuzzy set of young people can be described as follows.

F_young= { X, where 0<= μ (X)<=1 }

The graded membership μ of a person X to determine whether the person belongs to set of young people is defined as follows:

$\mu(X) = 1$ if age of X is > 0 years and <= 39 years

$\mu(X) = $ (age of X -60)/20 if age of X is > 39 years and <= 59 years

$\mu(X) = 0$ if age of X is > 59 years

Figure 1 describes various crisp and fuzzy sets for young people. Part (a) illustrates the crisp set having rigid partitions between young and old people. Part (b) illustrates a fuzzy set for young people. Part (c) describes alternative definitions of the fuzzy set for young people as such definitions are relative and vary person to person. Part (c) is comparatively smooth and gradual in nature. Such multiple definition of different fuzzy set sharing common universe can be defined in an integrated way as shown in Part (d). Image shown in Part (d) of Figure 1 describes 4 fuzzy sets which are described as Very Young, Young, Old and Very Old.

The possible candidates to the set defined in general are known as universe of discourse. The universe contains all elements that may be candidate of the set. For a fuzzy set, all the elements of the universe are members of the fuzzy set to some extent. For example, all people on the earth are members of the fuzzy set young people with different membership degree. Further, the fuzzy membership function to determine belongingness of an individual may be discrete or continuous.

Notion of the fuzzy membership functions helps in converting the crisp data into the fuzzy values by determining the fuzzy membership degree of a given element

Figure 1. Examples of a crisp set and fuzzy sets

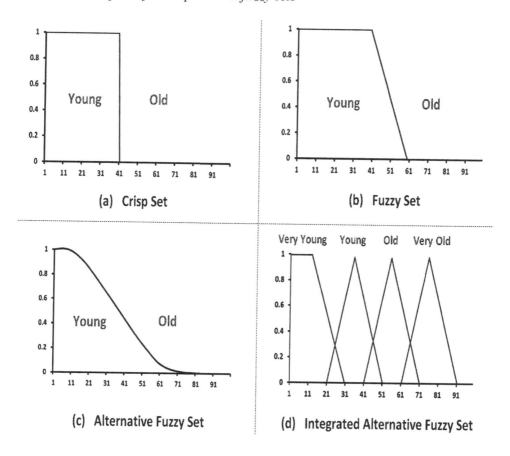

(a) Crisp Set

(b) Fuzzy Set

(c) Alternative Fuzzy Set

(d) Integrated Alternative Fuzzy Set

within the specific fuzzy set. However, at the lower level, the fuzzy data needs to be in the format which is machine operable. The same fuzzy membership function can be used as a guideline to achieve the appropriate crisp values via techniques called defuzzification. There are several defuzzification techniques available. Some of the most popular are center of gravity, mean of maxima and centroid methods.

Further, while considering the fuzzy set elements for decision making, one may consider linguistic variables associated with it. For the above example, linguistic variable 'Age' representing age of a person X may be defined. Possible values that the linguistic variable 'Age' can be 'Young', 'Very Young', 'Quite Young', 'Not Much Old', 'Old', etc. Such linguistic variables can be used in control structure such as rules. Examples of some fuzzy rules are given below.

- If Age of person is Young then assign the job A;

- If age of a person is Enough Old then assign desk job; etc.

Typical Boolean and relational operators as well as connectives can be used along with the fuzzy rules. Similarly, two fuzzy sets may be in relation with each other. A fuzzy rule may use more than one linguistic variables each corresponding to different fuzzy set. System which considers such rules and fuzzy sets is known as fuzzy logic based system. A rule base of such system hosts many fuzzy rules. In order to derive conclusions by applying rules from the system's rule base, one needs a mechanism that can produce an output from a collection of if-then-else type of rules. This is done using the mechanism of inference. It is also known as compositional rule of inference. A special control program for such system called an inference engine is developed. For a fuzzy logic based system, besides the rule base, an inference engine is one of the key components which play important roles. Figure 2 demonstrates the general structure showing other components of a typical fuzzy logic based system. An inference engine typically uses two main strategies to infer, which are called forward chaining and backward chaining. The forward chaining applies the available data to the suitable rules from the rule base in order to reach to the goal and completes the decision making process. In backward chaining, a hypothesis is made and compared in reverse manner to match the existing data.

The fuzzy logic based systems offer advantages of human like dealing with the systems and allows using loose as well as vague words as component of user's interactions with the system. Further, the fuzzy logic offers the more compact way to design rules which cover many situations in flexible way. Number of rules required to demonstrate the decision making situation are less in comparison with the traditional logic. In many consumer products, fuzzy logic is applied successfully. Fuzzy logic based decision making also have advantages of explanation and reasoning.

Figure 2. Components of a fuzzy logic based system

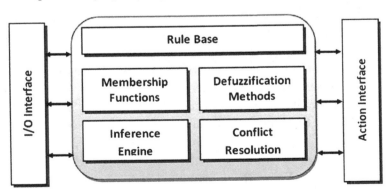

Inspite of attractive features and handsome benefits, the fuzzy logic based systems have no ability to learn from the data. There are many situations, where derivation of the generalised logic is difficult. In such cases, there is a need of technique that can learn some knowledge in absence of rules but with data. Artificial neural network is one of such technologies, which is described in next section.

Artificial Neural Network

Artificial Neural Network (ANN) is a technique that has its roots and inspiration from the Mother Nature. Human being can take intelligent and effective decisions using his nervous system. An artificial neural network can be considered as a simulation of human nervous system in a limited way. Such a network is collection of small, but large number of processing units working in parallel as well as asynchronous fashion. Each processing unit has little power, with which it can contribute towards a global solution. Such processing unit is called a neuron, which is a basic unit of the network. Being a pool of larger number of neurons having little proceeding capabilities, even if some of the neurons are not working; the system will still work. That is why such systems are fault tolerant.

There are many models available guiding us about the structure of neural network and how the learning process would take place. Following are some popular models of the artificial neural network.

- Hopfield network with parallel relaxation learning approach;
- Single and multiplayer perceptron with back propagation learning approach;
- Recurrent network, where connection between units are cyclic in nature;
- Kohonen model with unsupervised learning; etc.

The artificial neural network models can also be categorised according to the various learning paradigms such as supervised learning, unsupervised learning and reinforcement learning. In supervised leaning, training data sets are available. In unsupervised learning approach, network learns with the help of unlabeled data. In case of reinforcement learning, learning is done by interacting with environment.

The research work documented in this chapter uses fully connected multi-layer feed forward neural network with supervised learning paradigm. The general structure of the network is illustrated in Figure 3.

The perceptron learns in the following fashion.

- Designing the neural network phase
- Consider input parameters that are critical for decision making. Let these parameters be $X = \{x_1, x_2, x_3, ..., x_n\}$.

Figure 3. General structure of the multi-layer perceptron

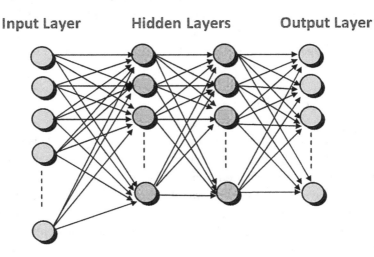

- Design an input layer with the above listed X with n neurons.
- Enlist the output opportunities. Let the set of all opportunities be $O = \{o_1, o_2, o_3, ..., o_m\}$.
- Design an output layer containing m neurons as denoted in the set O. Each output node has an output function.
- Consider two hidden layers. The number of nodes in the hidden layer may be considered as an (m+n)/2 ; where m is the total number of perceptron / nodes in the output layer and n is the total number of perceptron / nodes in the input layer. One may consider different heuristic. Each hidden node has hidden function within it.
- Connection phase
- Connect all the nodes of the network in such a way that each node is connected with every node of the immediate layer in forward direction only.
- Assign random weights to the connections.
- Learning phase
- Consider the first set of data. Give only input values to the input layers.
- Let your network computers what it thinks.
- Compare the output with the training set data output. Find out errors using the typical back propagation learning algorithm and adjust the weights. Repeat this till the network gives correct output for the data set or the error is acceptably small.
- Repeat the procedure for all the data sets.

This is a broad outline of supervised learning using back propagation learning paradigm. Since the network learns from the data, the quality of the neural network is directly dependent on the data. If data sets are poor and considers insignificant cases, the network learns to make decision as demonstrated in the data. Further, if data are good, but do not cover all categories of decision making examples, the neural network would be biased towards only given types of the data. When, in reality, new types of data are experienced, the network may not be able to provide correct output.

Such a network has many advantages. The main advantages include an ability to learn from the data in order to save time and effort; asynchronised and parallel control; and fault tolerance. However, the network is not able to document knowledge, as it is not having formal knowledge base. Knowledge is stored in the connections of a neural network, instead of formally documented in a knowledge base. Because of this reason, the neural network does not have an ability to explain its own decisions. To overcome this limitation, such network should be hybridised with other technologies. In next section, one such hybridization is discussed.

Neuro-Fuzzy Hybridization

The neuro-fuzzy hybridization incorporates two different methodology namely artificial neural network and fuzzy logic. As described in the previous section, the artificial neural network has limitations of explanation and reasoning, as the knowledge learned is documented in form of weights between the connections. The artificial neural network can learn from data and outputs accordingly to its learning. However, it can not document the generalised logic to solve the problem. Further, for future use and training as well as packing and selling (according to the intellectual property principles) of the documented knowledge is not available. On other hand, the fuzzy logic has very good ability to explain its own decision making using the documented knowledge within its knowledge base. If the fuzzy logic component is hybridised with an artificial neural network, it can overcome the limitations of the explanation and reasoning as well as it aids in dealing with the vague data and input from users. Vice versa, the fuzzy logic does not have an ability to learn from data, which can overcome by the neural network component. Such hybridization offers double advantages and overcome limitations of both the approaches.

The neuro-fuzzy hybridization can be employed in many ways. Some of the popular ways are as follows.

- Some components of the system use artificial neural network technology to perform assigned tasks to it. Other (one or more) components use fuzzy logic to compete its assigned tasks. Both these components work in cooperation of each other and communicate results to each another.

- Before assigning data to the artificial neural network, data can be acquired through a fuzzy interface allowing users to input vague and partial data. Such data can be defuzzified with the help of underlying membership functions returning crisp as well as normalized values as an ideal input to the neural network. Similarly, the neural network computes the required output, which is further converted into linguistic variables to be presented to the non-computer professionals. The fuzzy component can also be helpful in providing explanation to the users. Such work is demonstrated by Priti Srinivas Sajja and her colleagues (Trivedi & Sajja, 2011; Trivedi & Sajja, 2011; Sajja, 2011; Macwan & Sajja, 2014).

- The activation functions, output function and weights between the connections of a neural network may be fuzzy. Such work is demonstrated by Priti Srinivas Sajja and Jeegar Trivedi (Sajja & Trivedi, 2010). Instead of using the typical activation function, the neural network component may use application specific fuzzy activation function.

- The inference engine mechanism for a fuzzy logic component (such as backward chaining and forward chaining) as well as conflict resolution strategy can use artificial neural network to learn about the best possible fuzzy rules to be fired.

- The neural network component can also be used to derive fuzzy rules and suitable membership functions. Optionally, the rule evolution process can be strengthened by hybridizing one more component called genetic algorithm component (Mankad, Sajja, & Akerkar, 2011).

Besides the neuro-fuzzy hybridization, many bio-inspired models can be applicable for various advisory systems on the Web or semantic web. The detailed list and discussion is provided by Priti Srinivas Sajja and Rajendra Akerkar (2013). The work presented in this chapter uses neuro-fuzzy approach, which is described in next section.

GENERAL ARCHITECTURE OF NEURO-FUZZY SYSTEM

The experimental system for determination of customised nutrient requirements uses neuro-fuzzy hybrid approach. Underlying architecture of the system is generic in nature to support flexible use and multi domain functionality of the architecture. The architecture is shown in Figure 4.

Figure 4. Generic neuro-fuzzy architecture of the system

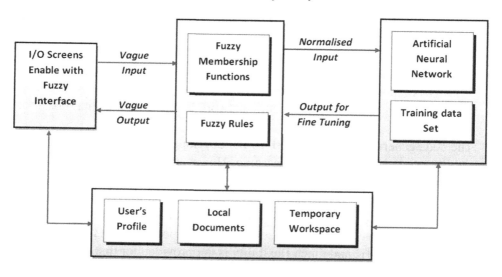

The architecture shown in Figure 4 has many major components. The first component is user interface. This user interface uses fuzzy logic as key technology. The basic aim of the fuzzy interface is to enable user to interact with the system in loose terms and vague inputs. The fuzzy words will be interpreted by appropriate fuzzy membership function and used by the fuzzy rules in the interface. Once proper course of action is deduced by the fuzzy rules and meaning of the vague input is made clear by the application of the fuzzy membership function, then equivalent machine understandable values are derived by the interface. These values are the normalised values for the neural network, working as the second component. The neural network is already trained artificial neural network. Here, we have used the multi layered feed forward fully connected perceptron. The number of nodes in the input layer, output layer and hidden layer can be changed as per the nature of the application by developers. The neural network outputs the results what it thinks. These results are in crisp format. Obviously, the users, who are non-computer professionals, desire the output of the system in much friendly way with added explanation. For this reasons, the generated output by the neural network is sent to the fuzzy interface, where it is converted into the text format for the benefit of users and presented on demand. It is to be noted that the architecture is generic in order to improve scope and usability of the architecture in various domains and applications. The code that generates the base artificial neural network is also flexible. It does the following tasks.

- It generates given number of input nodes in an input layer;
- It determines the number of hidden layers and nodes with the hidden layers by inbuilt heuristics,
- It generates output layer;
- It connects the nodes between the layers with feed forward connections and assigns random weights to them;
- On provision of data sets, the neural network learns from the data sets.

The code generates neural network by the developer's specifications and make it ready to use through supervised learning. However, the learning style remains supervisory. Similarly, the activation functions used in the neural network are also non-changeable. The flexibility is offered at two levels; at the time of number of nodes in input as well as output layers and at the provision of the training data sets. Similarly, the fuzzy membership functions and rules to be used in the fuzzy interface are application specific and much flexibility is not provided for that.

AN EXPERIMENT

With the advancement of computing infrastructure, expectations of people are also increasing. Sometimes highly ambitious expectations from users also encourage scientists and researchers for new inventions. Non computer professional expects help of computing technology more in their day to day lives. Daily nutrient requirements and advisory is one of such basic and trivial tasks. With the explosion of information on platforms like the Web, plenty of information available for common man; however, such information is really common and general and does not satisfy personal and customised needs. Such mundane tasks which look very simple and ordinary for human being are really complex for machines without intelligence. Beside advancements of technology, human living standard and activities have also been improved. These have increased stress and health problems. Many of the health problems can be weaken or overcome with the changed life style, proper diet plan and necessary exercises. With the help of typical database oriented computing infrastructure, it is difficult to provide personalised advisory about the nutrient requirement. The general information available on the websites may also be harmful to the individuals who may use it without complete knowledge.

Besides the domain knowledge, the system must know its users before presenting any advisory to them. For this reason, it is decided to use personalised neuro-fuzzy system to provide unique and customised advisory to its users. Using the neuro-fuzzy generic architecture discussed in the previous section of this chapter, an experimental system for determination of personal nutrient requirements is developed.

Fuzzy Interface

To provide advisory to the users the systems needs following basic inputs. These inputs are determined with help of domain experts, literature survey and according to the guidelines of the Health Level Seven International (HL7) (2014). The HL7 was founded in the year 1987. It is a non-profit organization that provides standards for the exchange, integration, sharing, and retrieval of electronic health information that supports clinical practice and the management, delivery and evaluation of health services. The input parameters are categorised into following categories.

- Personal parameters such as name, age, address and gender.

The field name and address are for the purpose of patient record in the database of the system, whereas the fields - age and gender are connected to intake of proper nutrients in diet. According to different age, there are different bodily requirement for nutrients. The gender also plays an important role in determination of nutrient requirement. Female need less intake of daily calorific food but they require more nutrients due to their metabolism. For example, iron is always necessary to increase haemoglobin level in blood in female. Hence, females are advised to take iron rich food items. The parameters age and gender are also utilized by fuzzy rule base to generate advice accordingly. The males are more likely to do physical work; hence total calorific requirement is higher than that of female. Hence, more nutrients are needed to carry out physical work due to requirement of more energy. Human body in itself is a science that converts nutrients taken as input to perform various day to day tasks. So it is easy to generalize that nutrients are fuel to human body. At different age, the need of nutrients increases or decreases from time to time. The exact age is calculated from date of birth field provided in the personal information fuzzy user interface.

To transfer the personal parameters input to the base neural network, the acquired input is calculated with following formula.

Personal_Info = Age/ 1000 + (Gender)

{Gender = 0.5 for Male & Gender = 0.4 for Female)

- Health related parameters such as height, weight and allergies.

From the parameters like height and weight body mass index is calculated automatically by the system. The body mass index is the basic parameter to determine the healthiness of a person. If body mass exceeds certain level than person is considered as obese and if it is less than certain level than the person is underweight. Furthermore, this category is also helpful in finding allergies that a person has. There are several type of allergies based on metabolism of individual. A person might be allergic to smell, medicine, dust and many other things. Human body can be hyper sensitive to allergic reaction that occur to it, hence proper care should be taken that the person is not exposed to allergic containing elements. Some element might be causing allergy in the person, for example some people are hypersensitive to medicine that contains sulphur as one of its ingredients, but sulphur is necessary nutrient required for the body. Hence, the system would advice to take diet in such a manner that sulphur is included as a part of nutritional value offered by the diet.

The formula to transfer the health related parameters input to the base neural network is given as follows.

Health = BMI – (Total Number of allergies)/10

{BMI = 0.8 if Normal Weight,

BMI = 0.5 if Over/Under Weight,

BMI = 0.3 if Obese}

• Parameters from the pathological reports.

The inputs are taken from reports like lipid profile, blood sugar level, blood pressure level and thyroid level in human body. These reports provide extremely vital information that directly affects functioning of human body. For example, if blood pressure is low then user is advised to take nutrients that are rich in salt contents, if blood pressure is high then user is advised to reduce salt intake. By taking proper nutrients these report values will automatically shift to their normal range. These parameters are also used by fuzzy rules in order to generate user specific advice. These input parameters are to be filled from respective medical reports of the person. In case where such reports are not available, the normal range is taken into consideration. However, it is advisable to go through various laboratory tests for exact insight of health of human body and need of nutrition to overcome the adverse conditions.

To transfer pathological parameter related input to the base neural network, following formula is used.

Report = (HDL/LDL) + (Sugar Level/1000) + (Systolic/Diastolic) + (Thyroid /1000)

For experiment purpose only the aforementioned pathological reports are considered. On inclusion of other parameters, the above formula should be modified.

• Routine dietary habits.

Some basic dietary and routine life style habits can have major impact in working of human body. Some habits like drinking alcohol or chewing tobacco can alter metabolic activities of human body. These habits adversely affect the bodily functions; hence more nutrition are needed to overcome deficiencies. For example, person chewing tobacco has reduced level of fat soluble vitamins like B1, B2, B6 and B12. Eating vegetarian food is a healthy habit, hence the system will advise, which habit to continue and which habit is required to be stopped.

Depending of the field survey parameters of different habits are determined and general formula is prepared as follows.

Habits $= 1 - \sum$(Habit per day)

{Continuously $= 0.008$,

More than thrice $= 0.006$,

Thrice $= 0.005$,

Twice $= 0.004$,

Once $= 0.002$}

The fuzzy membership function used for these parameters is given in Figure 5.

Table 1 represents Habit status with its fuzzy values and linguistic variable with triangular membership values.

Figure 6 represents a sample screen used to acquire habit related information. For each of the habit related parameters, a drop down list is presented to the users. Many of the habit related parameters are fuzzy in nature and each such fuzzy parameter use fuzzy membership function to obtain the equivalent crisp values as shown in Figure 6. For each category input, one or more screens are available, which are similar to the screen shown in Figure 6.

• Parameters related to family history:

Figure 5. Fuzzy membership functions for the habit parameter

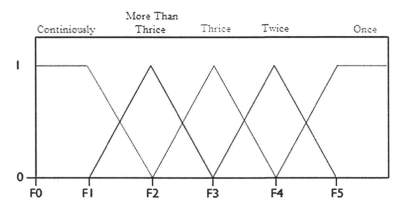

Table 1. Habit status with its fuzzy values

Linguistic Variable	Associated Fuzzy Number
Continuously	F0 = (1.0,0.9,0.8)
More than thrice	F1 = (0.8,0.8,0.7)
Thrice	F2 = (0.7,0.6,0.5)
Twice	F3 = (0.5,0.4,0.3)
Once	F4 = (0.3,0.2,0.1)

Figure 6. Input interface for acquiring habit related information

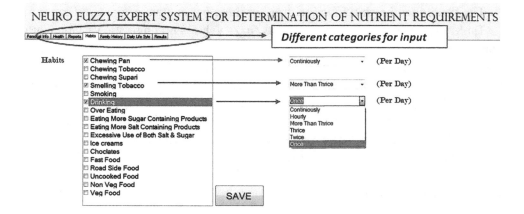

Such parameters provide information about family member's health status and the hereditary diseases. For example, if the user's ancestors suffered from heart problem then system will advice to reduce intake of food that are rich in fat contents, also it will advice to quit unhealthy habits, if any.

The family related fuzzy and non-fuzzy parameters are obtained via an interface screen and converted into a normalised value using following formula.

History = (accumulated crisp values obtained by membership functions) / 100

Figure 7 illustrates screen segment acquiring family history related information from users.

- Parameters related to the job profile:

These parameters provide information about daily life style of an individual user. Here, the lifestyle is categorized into three major categories of carrying out daily job of the user. The job may be totally physical like a labourer at construction site or moderately physical like data entry operators or totally nonphysical like IT professional. On the basis of their job category, different types of nutrients are es-

Figure 7. Screen segment acquiring family history related information

NEURO FUZZY EXPERT SYSTEM

| Personal Info | Health | Reports | Habits | Family History | Daily Life Syle | Results |

Family History

- ☑ Diabities
- ☐ Heart Problem
- ☐ Kideny Problem
- ☑ Neurological Problem
- ☐ Phycological Problem
- ☐ Hair Loss Problem
- ☐ Dry Skin Problem
- ☐ Haemophilia
- ☐ Victim of Nuclear Radiation
- ☐ Vision Problem
- ☐ Other Problem

SAVE

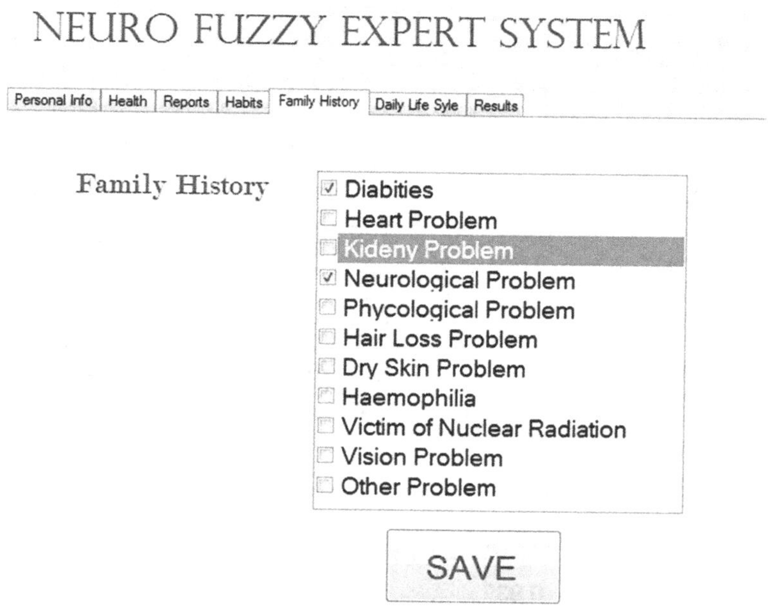

sential to survive in the existing job. For example, labourers prefer more jaggery related food items as their main diet, whereas wheat based diet for non labourers.

The normalised value for the job profile is calculated as follows.

Job_Profile = ((Job_Type) * (Total Number of Job)) / 100

Job_Type = {Physical = 0.008, Moderately Physical = 0.006, Non Physical = 0.004)

It is to be noted that the minimum value is 0 and maximum value is 1. If no data is available, then by default value 0.5 is passed to ANN.

Base Artificial Neural Network for the Experimental System

From the fuzzy interface six different normalised values are calculated as illustrated in the previous section. These values are normalised values for the artificial neural network input. The artificial neural network consists of an input layer consisting of six input neurons, two hidden layers having six neurons each and an output layer having three neurons. The simulated structure of the artificial neural network using JavaNNS (2014) is given as Figure 8.

Figure 8. Actual neural network for the experimental system

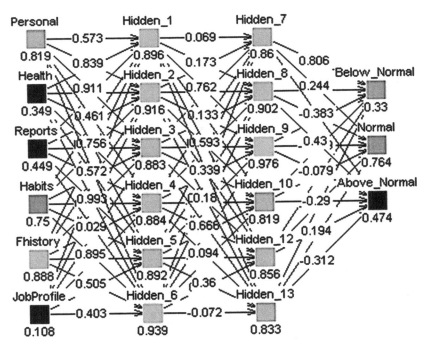

Output of the neural network is further just a value. The neural network classifies the users into three broad categories such as 'Above Normal', 'Normal', and 'Below Normal'. Such broad categories can be many depending on applications. The output of the neural network is passed to the output interface, which fine tunes the output and adds detailed advisory for better understanding of the output. See the following code snippet.

```
If (Output_Broad_Category == Above Normal)
{ If (Habit == Chewing Tobacco) && (Age > 40)
{Result += The person has low level of vitaminB  group due to
his dietary habit and routine
   lifestyle. The person is having higher chances of getting
beriberi. }
else if (Habit == Alcohol) && (Age >40)
{Result += The person can have alcoholic brain disease or heart
disease or Skin disorders,
   digestive problems. }
Result += The person is advised to take vitamin B rich nutrient
in his diet.
}
```

An output screen is shown in Figure 9.

Figure 9. An output interface generating final advisory

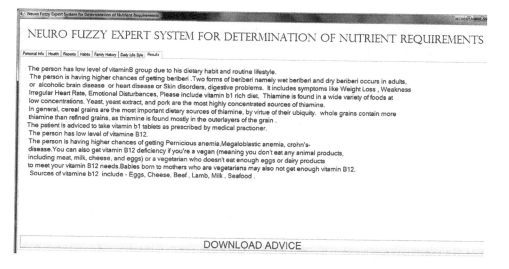

To convert the neural network output in user understandable and linguistic way, coding has been done. A sample code snippet is given below.

```
if (Gender == Male)
{If(age <40)
{ Personal_info = 0.8 }
        else If (age >= 40 && age <= 59)
        {Personal_info = 0.5}
else
      {Personal_info = 0.2}
}
else
{If(age <40)
{Personal_info = 0.7}
        else If (age >= 40 && age <= 59)
        {Personal_info = 0.5}
else
{Personal_info = 0.3}
}
```

Similarly, the values for other parameters are passed to artificial neural network with the help of encoding.

CONCLUSION

The experiment described in this chapter has advantages over typical IT based solutions. The prime advantages of the system are discussed here.

It has been observed that many good systems with best infrastructure fail because of acceptability and scope. Users generally confused with highly technical and rigid presentations and interface of the system. In the case of the proposed experimental system, the system interacts with the user as if expert is talking friendly to them. Such interaction of users with the system is facilitated in both the ways; at the time of information acquisition and while presenting system decision and advisory to the users.

The neural network learns from the successful cases through the data set provided for training. It has encoded knowledge of the past successful case histories in order to make correct and effective decision for the given inputs. The neural network cannot document the knowledge for future use and training, neither the network can provide detailed explanations to the decision take. This limitation can overcome with the component of interface enabling fuzzy logic for linguistic content representation.

The proposed structure of the neuro-fuzzy system is generic in nature and can be used in multiple domains with minor changes. Example domains are student's aptitude testing at various level, diagnosing and fault finding systems. The base neural network code as well as back propagation learning algorithm generated here are not application specific. However, the input – output fuzzy interface is application specific. Further, the membership functions are very specific and need to be developed according to the parameters selected.

In future a visual editor can be developed, especially for developers, which facilitates automatic generation of neuro-fuzzy systems in various domains. This can be considered as a commercial product and/or tool to generate soft computing based system.

REFERENCES

Bakker, I., Twisk, J. W., Mechelen, W., Menisink, G. B., & Kemper, H. C. (2003). Computerization of a dietary history interview in a running cohort; evaluation within the Amsterdam growth and health longitudinal study. *European Journal of Clinical Nutrition*, 57(3), 394–404. doi:10.1038/sj.ejcn.1601566 PMID:12627174

Bueche, J., Chamey, P., Pavlinac, J., Skipper, A., Thompson, A., & Myers, E. et al.. (2008). Nutrition care process and model part I: The 2008 update. *Journal of the American Dietetic Association*, 108(7), 1113–1117. doi:10.1016/j.jada.2008.04.027 PMID:18589014

Dwyer, J., Picciano, M. F., & Raiten, D. J. (2003). Future directions for the integrated CSFII-NHANES: What we eat in America-NHANES. *The Journal of Nutrition*, 133(2), 576S–581S. PMID:12566506

Engle, A., Lynn, L. L., Koury, K., & Boyar, A. P. (1990). Reproducibility and comparability of a computerized, self-administered food frequency questionnaire. *Nutrition and Cancer*, 13(4), 281–292. doi:10.1080/01635589009514070 PMID:2345706

Fahmi, A., Dorostanian, A., Rezazadeh, H., & Ostadrahimimi, A. (2013). An intelligent decision support system IDSS for nutrition therapy: Infrastructure, decision support, and knowledge management design. *International Journal of Reliable and Quality E-Healthcare*, 2(4), 14–27. doi:10.4018/ijrqeh.2013100102

Feskanich, D., Sielaff, B. H., Chong, K., & Buzzard, I. M. (1989). Computerized collection and analysis of dietary intake information. *Computer Methods and Programs in Biomedicine, 30*(1), 47–57. doi:10.1016/0169-2607(89)90122-3 PMID:2582746

Fong, A. K., & Kretsch, M. J. (1990). Nutrition evaluation scale system reduces time and labor in recording quantitative dietary intake. *Journal of the American Dietetic Association, 90*(5), 664–670. PMID:2335680

Frank, G. C. (1985). Nutrient profile on personal computers - a comparison of DINE with mainframe computers. *Health Education, 16*(1), 16–19. PMID:3939872

Gould, S. M., & Anderson, J. (2000). Using interactive multimedia nutrition education to reach low-income persons: An effective evaluation. *Journal of Nutrition Education, 32*(4), 204–213. doi:10.1016/S0022-3182(00)70558-9

Guthrie, H. A. (1989). Interpretation of data on dietary intake. *Nutrition Reviews, 47*(2), 33–38. doi:10.1111/j.1753-4887.1989.tb02780.x PMID:2654766

Health Level Seven International. (2014, December 19). *Health Level Seven International Home Page.* Retrieved December 19, 2014, from Health Level Seven International Web Site: http://www.hl7.org/

Hoggle, L. B., Michael, M. A., Houston, S. M., & Ayres, E. J. (2006). Nutrition informatics. *Journal of the American Dietetic Association, 106*(1), 134–139. doi:10.1016/j.jada.2005.10.025 PMID:16390678

Java, N. N. S. (2014, December 19). *Java NNS.* Retrieved December 19, 2014, from Java NNS Website: http://www.ra.cs.uni-tuebingen.de/software/JavaNNS/

Levine, J. A., Madden, A. M., & Morgan, M. Y. (1987). Validation of a computer based system for assessing dietary intake. *British Medical Journal (Clinical Research Ed.), 295*(6594), 369–372. doi:10.1136/bmj.295.6594.369 PMID:3115455

Macwan, N. A., & Sajja, P. S. (2014). Fuzzy logic: An effective user interface tool for decision support system. *International Journal of Engineering Science and Innovative Technology, 3*(3), 278–283.

Maillet, J. O., Skates, J., & Pritchett, E. (2005). American Dietetic Association: Scope of dietetics practice framework. *Journal of the American Dietetic Association, 105*(4), 634–640. doi:10.1016/j.jada.2005.02.001 PMID:15800568

Mankad, K. B., Sajja, P. S., & Akerkar, R. A. (2011). Evolving rules using genetic fuzzy approach - An educational case study. *International Journal on Soft Computing*, *2*(1), 35–46. doi:10.5121/ijsc.2011.2104

Nutrabalance Home Page. (2014, December 19). Retrieved December 19, 2014, from Nutrabalance Web Site: http://www.nutrabalance.com/

Probst, Y. C., & Tapsell, L. C. (2005). Overview of computerized dietary assessment programs for research and practice in nutrition education. *Journal of Nutrition Education and Behavior*, *37*(1), 20–26. doi:10.1016/S1499-4046(06)60255-8 PMID:15745652

Sajja, P. S. (2011). Personalized content representation through hybridization of mobile agent and interface agent. In S. Bagchi & S. Bagchi (Eds.), *Ubiquitous Multimedia and Mobile Agents: Models and Implementations* (pp. 85–112). Hershey, PA: IGI Global Book Publishing.

Sajja, P. S., & Akerkar, R. (2013). Bio-inspired models and the semantic web. In Z. C. Xin-She Yang & Z. C. Xin-She Yang (Eds.), *Swarm Intelligence and Bio-Inspired Computation: Theory and Applications* (pp. 273–294). Waltham, MA: Elsevier. doi:10.1016/B978-0-12-405163-8.00012-0

Sajja, P. S., & Trivedi, J. (2010). Using type-2 hyperbolic tangent activation function in artificial neural network. *Research Lines*, *3*(2), 51–57.

Sandström, B. (2001). A framework for food-based dietary guidelines in the European Union. *Public Health Nutrition*, *4*(2A), 293–305. PMID:11688435

Stein, K. (2010). Nutrition beyond the numbers: Counseling clients on nutrient value interpretation. *Journal of the Academy of Nutrition and Dietetics*, *110*(12), 1800–1803. PMID:21111084

Trivedi, J. A., & Sajja, P. S. (2011). Improving efficiency of round robin scheduling using neuro fuzzy approach. *International Journal of Research and Reviews in Computer Science*, *2*(2), 308–311.

Trivedi, J. A., & Sajja, P. S. (2011). Online guidance for effective investment using type-2 fuzzy neuro advisory system. *International Journal of Computer Science and Information Technologies*, *2*(2), 799–803.

Zadeh, L. A. (1965). Fuzzy sets. *Information and Control*, *8*(3), 338–353. doi:10.1016/S0019-9958(65)90241-X

KEY TERMS AND DEFINITIONS

Advisory System: An advisory system that provides advisory and decisions to its users. Such advisory systems interact with the users and also provide detailed explanation of the decision in form of explanation.

Artificial Neural Network: It is computer architecture inspired from the human nervous system. It can be considered as simulation of human nervous system in a very limited way. An artificial neural network contains large number of processing units called neurons, working in parallel and asynchronous way. Such artificial neural network has an ability to learn from data.

Back Propagation: Back propagation is defined as "backward propagation of errors". It is a common method of training artificial neural networks used in conjunction with an optimization method such as gradient descent.

Defuzzification Techniques: It is a technique to convert given fuzzy value into appropriate crisp values. There are several defuzzification techniques available. Some of the most popular are center of gravity, mean of maxima and centroid methods.

Fuzzy Logic: Fuzzy logic is multi valued logic allowing graded membership (rather than usual binary values such as 'true' or 'false', but between these values) of an entity to a class whose boundary is not defined. Such a class is known as fuzzy class.

Membership Functions: Membership functions (MFs) are the building blocks of fuzzy set theory. The degree of the membership of a given entity is determined through its corresponding membership function. Notion of the fuzzy membership functions helps in converting the crisp data into the fuzzy values by determining the fuzzy membership degree of a given element within the specific fuzzy set.

Neuro-Fuzzy System: The neuro-fuzzy hybridization incorporates two different methodology namely artificial neural network and fuzzy logic. A system based on such approach is called neuro-fuzzy system.

Supervised Learning: Supervised learning is the machine learning task of inferring a function from labelled training data. The training data consist of a set of training examples along with input as well as output.

Training Set: The training data set is a set of interrelated data with input and output (or questions with answers) for desirable cases in order to make the machine learn from it. Quality of the neural network learning depends on the training data set provided to it.

Compilation of References

Abowd, G. D., Dey, A. K., Brown, P. J., Davies, N., Smith, M., & Steggles, P. (1999). Towards a better understanding of context and context-awareness. In *1st International Symposium on Handheld and Ubiquitous Computing*. doi:10.1007/3-540-48157-5_29

Abu-Faraj, Z. O., Akar, H. A., Assaf, E. H., Al-Qadiri, M. N., & Youssef, E. G. (2010). Evaluation of fall and fall recovery in a simulated seismic environment: A pilot study. In *Proceedings of the EEE Annual International Conference of the IEngineering in Medicine and Biology Society (EMBC'10)*. doi:10.1109/IEMBS.2010.5627696

Acampora, G., Cook, D. J., Rashidi, P., & Vasilakos, A. V. (2013). A survey on ambient intelligence in healthcare. *Proceedings of the IEEE, 101*(12), 2470–2494. doi:10.1109/JPROC.2013.2262913 PMID:24431472

Acharya, R., Bhat, P. S., Kumar, S., & Min, L. C. (2003). Transmission and storage of medical images with patient information. *Computers in Biology and Medicine, 33*(4), 303–310. doi:10.1016/S0010-4825(02)00083-5 PMID:12791403

Ahlqvist, T., Bäck, A., Halonen, M., & Heinonen, S. (2008). Social media road maps exploring the futures triggered by social media. *VTT Tiedotteita - Valtion Teknillinen Tutkimuskeskus*, (2454), 13.

Ahmed, S., & Raja, M. (2010, December). Tackling cloud security issues and forensics model. In High-Capacity Optical Networks and Enabling Technologies (HONET), 2010 (pp. 190-195). IEEE. doi:10.1109/HONET.2010.5715771

Alagöz, F., Calero Valdez, A., Wilkowska, W., Ziefle, M., Dorner, S., & Holzinger, A. (2010). From cloud computing to mobile Internet, from user focus to culture and hedonism: The crucible of mobile health care and Wellness applications. In *Proceedings of 5th International Conference on Pervasive Computing and Applications (ICPCA'10)*. doi:10.1109/ICPCA.2010.5704072

Alamri, A., Ansari, W. S., Hassan, M. M., Hossain, M. S., Alelaiwi, A., & Hossain, M. A. (2013). A survey on sensor-cloud: Architecture, applications, and approaches. *International Journal of Distributed Sensor Networks, 2013*, 1–18. doi:10.1155/2013/917923

Alecsandru, R., Pruehsner, W., & Enderle, J. D. (1999). Remote Environmental Controller. In *Proceedings of the IEEE 25ᵗʰ Annual Northeast Bioengineering Conference*. IEEE.

Alemdar, H., & Ersoy, C. (2010). Wireless sensor networks for healthcare: A survey. *Computer Networks*, *54*(15), 2688–2710. doi:10.1016/j.comnet.2010.05.003

Alicja Muras, J., Cahill, V., & Katherine Stokes, E. (2006). A toxonomy of pervasive healthcare systems. In Pervasive Health Conference and Workshops.

Al-Jaroodi, J., & Mohamed, N. (2012). Service-oriented middleware: A survey. *Journal of Network and Computer Applications*, *35*(1), 211–220. doi:10.1016/j.jnca.2011.07.013

Alsafasfeh, Q. H., & Arfoa, A. A. (2011). Image encryption based on the general approach for multiple chaotic systems. *Journal of Signal and Information Processing*, *2*(03), 238–244. doi:10.4236/jsip.2011.23033

An Efficient Framework and Access Control Scheme for Cloud Health Care. (2015). In *Proceedings ofIEEE 7th International Conference on Cloud Computing Technology and Science (CloudCom)*. Vancouver, Canada: IEEE.

Anderson, D., Luke, R. H., Keller, J. M., Skubic, M., Rantz, M., & Aud, M. (2009). Linguistic summarization of video for fall detection using voxel person and fuzzy logic. *Computer Vision and Image Understanding*, *113*(1), 80–89. doi:10.1016/j.cviu.2008.07.006 PMID:20046216

Azodolmolky, S. (2013). *Software Defined Networking with OpenFlow*. Packt Publishing Ltd.

Bagala, F., Becker, C., Cappello, A., Chiari, L., Aminian, K., Hausdorff, J. M., & Klenk, J. et al. (2012). Evaluation of accelerometer-based fall detection algorithms on real-world falls. *PLoS ONE*, *7*(5), 1–9. doi:10.1371/journal.pone.0037062 PMID:22615890

Bakker, I., Twisk, J. W., Mechelen, W., Menisink, G. B., & Kemper, H. C. (2003). Computerization of a dietary history interview in a running cohort; evaluation within the Amsterdam growth and health longitudinal study. *European Journal of Clinical Nutrition*, *57*(3), 394–404. doi:10.1038/sj.ejcn.1601566 PMID:12627174

Balamurugan, B., Krishna, P. V., Rajya Lakshmi, G. V., & Kumar, N. S. (2014, July). Cloud cluster communication for critical applications accessing C-MPICH. In *Embedded Systems (ICES), 2014 International Conference on* (pp. 145-150). IEEE.

Balamurugan, B., Venkata Krishna, P., Rajya, L. G., & Saravana Kumar, N. (2014, May). Layered storage architecture for health system using cloud. In *Advanced Communication Control and Computing Technologies (ICACCCT), 2014 International Conference on* (pp. 1795-1800). IEEE. doi:10.1109/ICACCCT.2014.7019419

Balamurugan, B., Krishna, P. V., Kumar, N. S., & Rajyalakshmi, G. V. (2015). An Efficient Framework for Health System Based on Hybrid Cloud with ABE-Outsourced Decryption. In *Artificial Intelligence and Evolutionary Algorithms in Engineering Systems* (pp. 41–49). Springer India. doi:10.1007/978-81-322-2135-7_6

Balamurugan, B., Kumar, N. S., Lakshmi, G. V., & Shanmuga, R. N. S. (2014, November). Common Cloud Architecture for Cloud Interoperability. In *Proceedings of the 2014 International Conference on Information and Communication Technology for Competitive Strategies* (p. 10). ACM.

Balamurugan, B., & Kumar, S. (2013). Enhancing privacy in cloud using Attribute Based Encryption. In *International Conference on Mathematical Computer Engineering-ICMCE* (p. 641).

Bali, R., Troshani, I., & Wickramasinghe, N. (2013). *Pervasive Health Knowledge Management*. Springer. doi:10.1007/978-1-4614-4514-2

Bamiah, M., Brohi, S., & Chuprat, S. (2012). A study on significance of adopting cloud computing paradigm in healthcare sector. In *International Conference on Cloud Computing, Technologies, Applications & Management*. doi:10.1109/ICCCTAM.2012.6488073

Best, J. (2011). IBM Watson the Inside Story. *Tech Republic*. Retrieved January 21, 2016, from http://www.techrepublic.com/article/ibm-watson-the-inside-story-of-how-the-jeopardy-winning-supercomputer-was-born-and-what-it-wants-to-do-next/

Bethencourt, J., Sahai, A., & Waters, B. (2007). Ciphertext-policy attributebased encryption. In *Security and Privacy, SP '07. IEEE Symposium on*, (pp. 321–334). IEEE.

Betke, M., Gips, J., & Fleming, P. (2002). The camera mouse: Visual tracking of body features to provide computer access for people with severe disabilities. *IEEE Transactions on Neural Systems and Rehabilitation Engineering*, *10*(1), 1–10. doi:10.1109/TNSRE.2002.1021581 PMID:12173734

Bianchi, F., Redmond, S. J., Narayanan, M. R., Cerutti, S., & Lovell, N. H. (2010). Barometric pressure and triaxial accelerometry-based falls event detection. *IEEE Transactions on Neural Systems and Rehabilitation Engineering*, *18*(6), 619–627. doi:10.1109/TNSRE.2010.2070807 PMID:20805056

Biswas, J., Jayachandran, M., Shue, L., Gopalakrishnan, K., & Yap, P. (2009). *Design and trial deployment of a practical sleep activity pattern monitoring system. In Ambient Assistive Health and Wellness Management in the Heart of the City* (pp. 190–200). Springer.

Bohonos, S., Lee, A., Malik, A., Thai, C., & Manduchi, R. (2007). Universal real-time navigational assistance (URNA): an urban bluetooth beacon for the blind. In *Proceedings of the 1st ACM international workshop on Systems and networking support for healthcare and assisted living environments (SIGMOBILE'07)*. doi:10.1145/1248054.1248080

Bottles, K., & Begoli, E. (2014). Understanding the pros and cons of big data analytics. *Physician Executive*, *40*, 6–12. PMID:25188972

Boughzala, B., Ben Ali, R., Lemay, M., Lemieux, Y., & Cherkaoui, O. (2011, May). OpenFlow supporting inter-domain virtual machine migration. In *Wireless and Optical Communications Networks (WOCN), 2011 Eighth International Conference on* (pp. 1-7). IEEE. doi:10.1109/WOCN.2011.5872945

Bourke, A. K., O'Brien, J. V., & Lyons, G. M. (2007). Evaluation of a threshold-based tri-axial accelerometer fall detection algorithm. *Gait & Posture*, *26*(2), 194–199. doi:10.1016/j.gaitpost.2006.09.012 PMID:17101272

Bourke, A. K., van de Ven, P., Gamble, M., O'Connor, R., Murphy, K., Bogan, E., & Nelson, J. et al. (2010). Assessment of waist-worn tri-axial accelerometer based fall-detection algorithms using continuous unsupervised activities. In *Proceedings of IEEE Annual International Conference of the Engineering in Medicine and Biology Society (EMBC'10)*. doi:10.1109/IEMBS.2010.5626364

Bouslimi, D., Coatrieux, G., Cozic, M., & Roux, C. (2012). A joint encryption/watermarking system for verifying the reliability of medical images. *Information Technology in Biomedicine. IEEE Transactions on*, *16*(5), 891–899.

Brunette, G., & Mogull, R. (2009). Security guidance for critical areas of focus in cloud computing v2. 1. *Cloud Security Alliance*, 1-76..

Bueche, J., Chamey, P., Pavlinac, J., Skipper, A., Thompson, A., & Myers, E. et al.. (2008). Nutrition care process and model part I: The 2008 update. *Journal of the American Dietetic Association*, *108*(7), 1113–1117. doi:10.1016/j.jada.2008.04.027 PMID:18589014

Candemir, S., Jaeger, S., Palaniappan, K., Musco, J. P., Singh, R. K., Xue, Z., & McDonald, C. J. et al. (2014). Lung segmentation in chest radiographs using anatomical atlases with nonrigid registration. *IEEE Transactions on Medical Imaging*, *33*(2), 577–590. doi:10.1109/TMI.2013.2290491 PMID:24239990

Celik, M. U., Sharma, G., & Saber, E. (2002). Reversible data hiding. In *Image Processing. 2002. Proceedings. 2002 International Conference on* (Vol. 2, pp. II-157). IEEE. doi:10.1109/ICIP.2002.1039911

Chawla, N. V., & Davis, D. A. (2013). Bringing *big data to personalized healthcare: A patient-centered framework*. *Journal of General Internal Medicine*, *28*(S3), S660–S665. doi:10.1007/s11606-013-2455-8 PMID:23797912

Chen, J., Kwong, K., Chang, D., Luk, J., & Bajcsy, R. (2006). Wearable sensors for reliable fall detection. In *Proceedings of the 27ᵗʰ Annual International Conference of the Engineering in Medicine and Biology Society* (IEEE-EMBS'05). doi:10.1109/IEMBS.2005.1617246

Chen, H. C., Chiang, R. H. L., & Storey, V. C. (2012). Business intelligence and analytics: From big data to big impact. *Management Information Systems Quarterly, 36*, 1165–1188.

Chen, Y.-L. (2001). Application of tilt sensors in human-computer mouse interface for people with disabilities. *IEEE Transactions on Neural Systems and Rehabilitation Engineering, 9*(3), 289–294. doi:10.1109/7333.948457 PMID:11561665

Cheung, Y. M., & Wu, H. T. (2007). A sequential quantization strategy for data embedding and integrity verification. *Circuits and Systems for Video Technology. IEEE Transactions on, 17*(8), 1007–1016.

Chorafas, D. (2011). *Cloud Computing Strategies*. Taylor and Francis Group, LLC.

Chuah, M., & DiBlasio, M. (2012). Smartphone based autism social alert system. In *Proceedings of the 8th International Conference on Mobile Ad-hoc and Sensor Networks (MSN'12)*.

Cloud Security Alliance. (2011). *STAR (security, trust and assurance registry) program*. doi:10.1007/978-3-642-29852-3_7

Coatrieux, G., Maitre, H., Sankur, B., Rolland, Y., & Collorec, R. (2000). Relevance of watermarking in medical imaging. In *Information Technology Applications in Biomedicine, 2000. Proceedings. 2000 IEEE EMBS International Conference on* (pp. 250-255). IEEE. doi:10.1109/ITAB.2000.892396

Coatrieux, G., Le Guillou, C., Cauvin, J. M., & Roux, C. (2009). Reversible watermarking for knowledge digest embedding and reliability control in medical images. *Information Technology in Biomedicine. IEEE Transactions on, 13*(2), 158–165.

Coronato, A., De Pietro, G., & Sannino, G. (2010). Middleware services for pervasive monitoring elderly and ill people in smart environments. In *Seventh International Conference on Information Technology*. doi:10.1109/ITNG.2010.139

Corredor, I., Tarrio, P., Bernardos, A. M., & Casar, J. R. (2013). An open architecture to enhance pervasiveness and mobility of health care services. *Communications in Computer and Information Science, 413*, 296–307. doi:10.1007/978-3-319-04406-4_30

Cote, R. A. (1986, October). Architecture of SNOMED: its contribution to medical language processing. In *Proceedings of the Annual Symposium on Computer Application in Medical Care* (p. 74). American Medical Informatics Association.

Coughlan, J., & Manduchi, R. (2007). Color targets: Fiducials to help visually impaired people find their way by camera phone. *EURASIP Journal on Image and Video Processing*.

Cox, I. J., Kilian, J., Leighton, F. T., & Shamoon, T. (1997). Secure spread spectrum watermarking for multimedia. *Image Processing. IEEE Transactions on*, *6*(12), 1673–1687.

Cox, I. J., Miller, M. L., Bloom, J. A., & Honsinger, C. (2002). *Digital watermarking* (Vol. 53). San Francisco: Morgan Kaufmann.

Cox, I., Miller, M., Bloom, J., Fridrich, J., & Kalker, T. (2007). *Digital watermarking and steganography*. Morgan Kaufmann.

Cucchiara, R., Prati, A., & Vezzani, R. (2007). A multi-camera vision system for fall detection and alarm generation. *Expert Systems: International Journal of Knowledge Engineering and Neural Networks*, *24*(5), 334–345. doi:10.1111/j.1468-0394.2007.00438.x

De Vleeschouwer, C., & Macq, B. (2003). Circular interpretation of bijective transformations in lossless watermarking for media asset management. *Multimedia. IEEE Transactions on*, *5*(1), 97–105.

Debroha, D. (2015). IBM Watson Health Announces New Partnership. *IBM PR Newswire*. Retrieved January 20, 2016, from http://www.prnewswire.com/news/ibm+watson+health

Demiris, G., Hensel, B., Skubic, M., & Rantz, M. (2008). Senior residents' perceived need of and preferences for``smart home''sensor technologies. *International Journal of Technology Assessment in Health Care*, *24*(1), 120–124. doi:10.1017/S0266462307080154 PMID:18218177

Diffie, W., & Hellman, M. E. (1976). New directions in cryptography. *Information Theory. IEEE Transactions on*, *22*(6), 644–654.

Dikaiakos, M. D., Katsaros, D., Mehra, P., Pallis, G., & Vakali, A. (2009). Cloud computing: Distributed internet computing for IT and scientific research. *IEEE Internet Computing*, *13*(5), 10–13. doi:10.1109/MIC.2009.103

Dillon, T., Wu, C., & Chang, E. (2010). Cloud Computing: Issues and Challenges. In *Proceedings of Advanced Information Networking and Applications (AINA), 2010 24th IEEE International Conference on.* doi:10.1201/9781439834541

Diraco, G., Leone, A., & Siciliano, P. (2010). An active vision system for fall detection and posture recognition in elderly healthcare. In *Proceedings of the Design, Automation & Test in Europe Conference & Exhibition* (DATE'10).

Dooley, J. (2012). *Intelligent Environments Group.* University of Essex. Retrieved 6 18, 2014, from http://iieg.essex.ac.uk/idorm.htm/

Doukas, C., & Maglogiannis, I. (2012). Bringing IoT and cloud computing towards pervasive healthcare. In Innovative Mobile and Internet Services in Ubiquitous Computing. doi:10.1109/IMIS.2012.26

Doukas, C., & Maglogiannis, I. (2011). Managing wearable sensor data through cloud computing. In *International Conference on Cloud Computing Technology and Science.* doi:10.1109/CloudCom.2011.65

Doukas, C., Pliakas, T., & Maglogiannis, I. (2010). Mobile healthcare information management utilizing Cloud Computing and Android OS. In *Proceedings of the IEEE Annual International Conference of the Engineering in Medicine and Biology Society (EMBC'10).* IEEE.

Dwyer, J., Picciano, M. F., & Raiten, D. J. (2003). Future directions for the integrated CSFII-NHANES: What we eat in America-NHANES. *The Journal of Nutrition, 133*(2), 576S–581S. PMID:12566506

Ekonomou, M., Fan, L., Buchanan, W., & Thuemmler, C. (2011). An Integerated Cloud-based Healthcare Infrastructure. In *Third IEEE International Conference on Cloud Computing Technology and Science.* doi:10.1109/CloudCom.2011.80

El Alamy, L., Lhaddad, S., Maalal, S., Taybi, Y., & Salih-Alj, Y. (2012). Bus Identification System for Visually Impaired Person. In *Proceedings of the 6th International Conference on Next Generation Mobile Applications, Services and Technologies (NGMAST'12).* doi:10.1109/NGMAST.2012.22

Engle, A., Lynn, L. L., Koury, K., & Boyar, A. P. (1990). Reproducibility and comparability of a computerized, self-administered food frequency questionnaire. *Nutrition and Cancer, 13*(4), 281–292. doi:10.1080/01635589009514070 PMID:2345706

European Network and Information Security Agency. (2009). *Cloud Computing: Benefits, risks and recommendations for information security.* ENISA.

F., C. (n.d.). Global Information Policymaking and Domestic Law. *Indiana Journal of Global Legal Studies,* 467-487.

Fahmi, A., Dorostanian, A., Rezazadeh, H., & Ostadrahimimi, A. (2013). An intelligent decision support system IDSS for nutrition therapy: Infrastructure, decision support, and knowledge management design. *International Journal of Reliable and Quality E-Healthcare, 2*(4), 14–27. doi:10.4018/ijrqeh.2013100102

Fan, L., Buchanan, W., Thuemmler, C., Lo, O., Khedim, A., Uthmani, O., . . . Bell, D. (2011, July). DACAR platform for eHealth services cloud. In *Cloud Computing (CLOUD), 2011 IEEE International Conference on* (pp. 219-226). IEEE. doi:10.1109/CLOUD.2011.31

Fan, L., Buchanan, W., Thummler, C., Lo, O., Khedim, A., Uthmani, O., & Bell, D. et al. (2011). DACAR Platform for eHealth Services Cloud. In *Proceedings of the IEEE International Conference on Cloud Computing (CLOUD'11).*

Feldman, S., & Handover, J. (2012). Unlocking the Power of Unstructured Data. *IDC Health Insights.* Retrieved January 21, 2016, from http:/www01.ibm.com/software/ebusiness/jstart /downloads/unlockingUnstructuredData.pdf

Fernández-Alemán, J. L., Señor, I. C., Lozoya, P. Á. O., & Toval, A. (2013). Security and privacy in electronic health records: A systematic literature review. *Journal of Biomedical Informatics, 46*(3), 541–562. doi:10.1016/j.jbi.2012.12.003 PMID:23305810

Feskanich, D., Sielaff, B. H., Chong, K., & Buzzard, I. M. (1989). Computerized collection and analysis of dietary intake information. *Computer Methods and Programs in Biomedicine, 30*(1), 47–57. doi:10.1016/0169-2607(89)90122-3 PMID:2582746

Fong, A. K., & Kretsch, M. J. (1990). Nutrition evaluation scale system reduces time and labor in recording quantitative dietary intake. *Journal of the American Dietetic Association, 90*(5), 664–670. PMID:2335680

Frank, G. C. (1985). Nutrient profile on personal computers - a comparison of DINE with mainframe computers. *Health Education, 16*(1), 16–19. PMID:3939872

Fridrich, J., Goljan, M., & Du, R. (2001, August). Invertible authentication. In Photonics West 2001-Electronic Imaging (pp. 197-208). International Society for Optics and Photonics.

Fu, Z., Delbruck, T., Lichtsteiner, P., & Culurciello, E. (2008). An address-event fall detector for assisted living applications. *IEEE Transactions on Biomedical Circuits and Systems*, 2(2), 88–96. doi:10.1109/TBCAS.2008.924448 PMID:23852755

Ganz, A., Schafer, J., Gandhi, S., Puleo, E., Wilson, C., & Robertson, M. (2012). PERCEPT indoor navigation system for the blind and visually impaired: Architecture and experimentation. *International Journal of Telemedicine and Applications*, 2012, 19. doi:10.1155/2012/894869 PMID:23316225

Goljan, M., Fridrich, J. J., & Du, R. (2001, January). Distortion-free data embedding for images. In *Information Hiding* (pp. 27–41). Springer Berlin Heidelberg. doi:10.1007/3-540-45496-9_3

Gould, S. M., & Anderson, J. (2000). Using interactive multimedia nutrition education to reach low-income persons: An effective evaluation. *Journal of Nutrition Education*, 32(4), 204–213. doi:10.1016/S0022-3182(00)70558-9

Guan, Z. H., Huang, F., & Guan, W. (2005). Chaos-based image encryption algorithm. *Physics Letters. [Part A]*, 346(1), 153–157. doi:10.1016/j.physleta.2005.08.006

Guide to Data Protection. (n.d.). Retrieved from https://ico.org.uk/for-organisations/guide-to-data-protection/

Guo, B., Sun, L., & Zhang, D. (2010). The Architecture Design of a Cross-Domain Context Management System. In *8th IEEE international conference on pervasive computing and communications workshops.* doi:10.1109/PERCOMW.2010.5470618

Guthrie, H. A. (1989). Interpretation of data on dietary intake. *Nutrition Reviews*, 47(2), 33–38. doi:10.1111/j.1753-4887.1989.tb02780.x PMID:2654766

Halamka, J. D. (2014). Early experiences with big data at an academic medical center. *Health Affairs*, 33(7), 1132–1138. doi:10.1377/hlthaff.2014.0031 PMID:25006138

Haq, I. U., Alnemr, R., Paschke, A., Schikuta, E., Boley, H., & Meinel, C. (2010). Distributed trust management for validating sla choreographies. In Grids and service-oriented architectures for service level agreements (pp. 45-55). Springer US. doi:10.1007/978-1-4419-7320-7_5

Hazelhoff, L., & Han, J. (2008). Video-based fall detection in the home using principal component analysis. In *Proceedings of the Advanced Concepts for Intelligent Vision Systems.* doi:10.1007/978-3-540-88458-3_27

Health Level Seven International. (2014, December 19). *Health Level Seven International Home Page*. Retrieved December 19, 2014, from Health Level Seven International Web Site: http://www.hl7.org/

Helal, A., Moore, S. E., & Ramachandran, B. (2001). Drishti: An integrated navigation system for visually impaired and disabled. In *Proceedings of the 5th International Symposium on Wearable Computers*. doi:10.1109/ISWC.2001.962119

Helm-Murtagh, S. C. (2014). Use of Big Data by Blue Cross and Blue Shield of North Carolina. *NCMJ*, *75*, 195–197. PMID:24830494

HIPPA. (1996). *Health Insurance Portability and Accountability Act of 1996 (HIPPA)*. Retrieved from: http://aspe.hhs.gov/admnsimp/pl104191.htm

Hoggle, L. B., Michael, M. A., Houston, S. M., & Ayres, E. J. (2006). Nutrition informatics. *Journal of the American Dietetic Association*, *106*(1), 134–139. doi:10.1016/j.jada.2005.10.025 PMID:16390678

Honsinger, C. W., Jones, P. W., Rabbani, M., & Stoffel, J. C. (2001). *U.S. Patent No. 6,278,791*. Washington, DC: U.S. Patent and Trademark Office.

Hossain, M. S., & Muhammad, G. (2014). Cloud-based collaborative media service framework for healthcare. *International Journal of Distributed Sensor Networks*, *2014*, 1–11.

Huang, J., & Nicol, D. M. (2013). Trust mechanisms for cloud computing. *Journal of Cloud Computing*, *2*(1), 1–14.

Igual, R., Medrano, C., & Plaza, I. (2013). Challenges, issues and trends in fall detection systems. *Biomedical Engineering Online*, *12*(1), 66–66. doi:10.1186/1475-925X-12-66 PMID:23829390

Imam Reza Specialized & Sub-Specialized Hospital. (n.d.). Retrieved 3 05, 2014, from http://www.imamreza.ajaums.ac.ir

Introduction to Biosensors. (n.d.). Retrieved from www.sirebi.org

Ismail, I. A., Amin, M., & Diab, H. (2010). A digital image encryption algorithm based a composition of two chaotic logistic maps. *International Journal of Network Security*, *11*(1), 1–10.

Jaeger, S., Karargyris, A., Candemir, S., Folio, L., Siegelman, J., Callaghan, F., & Thoma, G. et al. (2014). Automatic tuberculosis screening using chest radiographs. *IEEE Transactions on Medical Imaging*, *33*(2), 233–245. doi:10.1109/TMI.2013.2284099 PMID:24108713

Jansen, W., & Grance, T. (2011). Guidelines on security and privacy in public cloud computing. *NIST Special Publication, 800*(144), 10-11.

Jara, A. J., Zamora, M. A., & Skarmeta, A. F. G. (2011). An Internet of things-based personal device for diabetes therapy management in ambient assisted living (AAL). *Personal and Ubiquitous Computing, 15*(4), 431–440. doi:10.1007/s00779-010-0353-1

Java, N. N. S. (2014, December 19). *Java NNS*. Retrieved December 19, 2014, from Java NNS Website: http://www.ra.cs.uni-tuebingen.de/software/JavaNNS/

Jennings, R. (2009). *Cloud Computing with the Windows Azure Platform*. Wrox Press Ltd.

Jit, B., Maniyeri, J., Louis, S., & Philip, Y. L. K. (2009). *Fast matching of sensor data with manual observations*. Paper presented at the Annual International Conference of the IEEE Engineering in Medicine and Biology Society. doi:10.1109/IEMBS.2009.5333881

Juan, C., Xiang, C., & Minfen, S. (2013). A framework for daily activity monitoring and fall detection based on surface electromyography and accelerometer signals. *IEEE Journal of Biomedical and Health Informatics, 17*(1), 38-45.

Kafah, O., Bromuri, S., Sindlar, M., Weide, T., Aguilar Pelaez, E., Schaetchle, U., … Stathis, K. (2013). COMMODITY12: A smart e-health environment for diabetes management. *Journal of Ambient Intelligence and Smart Environments*, 479-502.

Kaletsch, A., & Sunyaev, A. (2011). *Privacy engineering: personal health records in cloud computing environments*. Academic Press.

Kangas, M., Konttila, A., Lindgren, P., Winblad, I., & Timo, J. (2008). Comparison of low-complexity fall detection algorithms for body attached accelerometers. *Gait & Posture, 28*(2), 285–291. doi:10.1016/j.gaitpost.2008.01.003 PMID:18294851

Kangas, M., Vikman, I., Wiklander, J., Lindgren, P., Nyberg, L., & Timo, J. (2009). Sensitivity and specificity of fall detection in people aged 40 years and over. *Gait & Posture, 29*(4), 571–574. doi:10.1016/j.gaitpost.2008.12.008 PMID:19153043

Khan, A., Siddiqa, A., Munib, S., & Malik, S. A. (2014). A recent survey of reversible watermarking techniques. *Information Sciences, 279*, 251–272. doi:10.1016/j.ins.2014.03.118

Kim, H., Kim, J., & Ko, Y. B. (2014, February). Developing a cost-effective OpenFlow-testbed for small-scale Software Defined Networking. In *Advanced Communication Technology (ICACT), 2014 16th International Conference on* (pp. 758-761). IEEE.

Krasij, A. B., Pruehsner, W., & Enderle, J. D. (1999). VoxyBox. In *Proceedings of the 25th IEEE Annual Northeast Bioengineering Conference*. doi:10.1109/NEBC.1999.755767

Krutz, R. L., & Vines, R. D. (2010). *Cloud security: A comprehensive guide to secure cloud computing*. Wiley Publishing.

Kumar, N. S., Lakshmi, G. R., & Balamurugan, B. (2015). Enhanced Attribute Based Encryption for Cloud Computing. *Procedia Computer Science*, *46*, 689–696. doi:10.1016/j.procs.2015.02.127

Kuo, A. M. H., Borycki, E., Kushniruk, A., & Lee, T. S. (2011). A healthcare Lean Six Sigma System for postanesthesia care unit workflow improvement. *Quality Management in Health Care*, *20*(1), 4–14. doi:10.1097/QMH.0b013e3182033791 PMID:21192203

Kupryjanow, A., Kunka, B., & Kostek, B. (2010). UPDRS Tests for Diagnosis of Parkinson's Disease Employing Virtual-Touchpad. In *Proceedings of the DEXA Workshops*. doi:10.1109/DEXA.2010.87

Lai, Deng, Guan, & Weng. (2013). Attribute-based encryption with verifiable outsourced decryption. *IEEE Transactions on Information Forensics and Security*, *8*(8), 1343–1354.

Lai, C.-F., Chang, S.-Y., Chao, H.-C., & Huang, Y.-M. (2011). Detection of cognitive injured body region using multiple tri-axial accelerometers for elderly falling. *IEEE Sensors Journal*, *11*(3), 763–770. doi:10.1109/JSEN.2010.2062501

Lakrissi, Y., Erritali, M., & Fakir, M. (2013). A Joint Encryption/Watermarking Algorithm for Secure Image Transfer. *International Journal of Computer Networking and Communication*, *1*(1). doi:10.1109/TCSVT.2015.2418611

Lantz, B., Heller, B., & McKeown, N. (2010, October). A network in a laptop: rapid prototyping for software-defined networks. In *Proceedings of the 9th ACM SIGCOMM Workshop on Hot Topics in Networks* (p. 19). ACM. doi:10.1145/1868447.1868466

Lara, A., Kolasani, A., & Ramamurthy, B. (2014). Network innovation using openflow: A survey. *IEEE Communications Surveys and Tutorials*, *16*(1), 493–512. doi:10.1109/SURV.2013.081313.00105

Le Bellego, G., Noury, N., Virone, G., Mousseau, M., & Demongeot, J. (2006). A model for the measurement of patient activity in a hospital suite. *Information Technology in Biomedicine,* 92-99.

Lee, K., Murray, D., Hughes, D., & Joosen, W. (2010). *Extending sensor networks into the cloud using amazon web services.* Paper presented at the IEEE International Conference on Networked Embedded Systems for Enterprise Applications (NESEA 2010). doi:10.1109/NESEA.2010.5678063

Lee, T., & Mihailidis, A. (2005). An intelligent emergency response system: Preliminary development and testing of automated fall detection. *Journal of Telemedicine and Telecare, 11*(4), 194–198. doi:10.1258/1357633054068946 PMID:15969795

Lee, Y.-B., & Lee, M.-H. (2009). Indoor Positioning System for Moving Objects on an Indoor for Blind or Visually Impaired Playing Various Sports. *Proceedings of Journal of Electrical Engineering And Technology, 4*(1), 131–134. doi:10.5370/JEET.2009.4.1.131

LeMoyne, R., Coroian, C., & Mastroianni, T. (2009). Quantification of Parkinson's disease characteristics using wireless accelerometers. In *Proceedings of International Conference on Complex Medical Engineering (ICME'09).* doi:10.1109/ICCME.2009.4906657

LeMoyne, R., Mastroianni, T., Cozza, M., Coroian, C., & Grundfest, W. (2010). Implementation of an iPhone for characterizing Parkinson's disease tremor through a wireless accelerometer application. In *Proceedings of IEEE Annual International Conference of the Engineering in Medicine and Biology Society (EMBC'10).* doi:10.1109/IEMBS.2010.5627240

Levine, J. A., Madden, A. M., & Morgan, M. Y. (1987). Validation of a computer based system for assessing dietary intake. *British Medical Journal (Clinical Research Ed.), 295*(6594), 369–372. doi:10.1136/bmj.295.6594.369 PMID:3115455

Levoy, M., Pulli, K., Curless, B., Rusinkiewicz, S., Koller, D., Pereira, L., & Fulk, D. et al. (2000, July). The digital Michelangelo project: 3D scanning of large statues. In *Proceedings of the 27th annual conference on Computer graphics and interactive techniques* (pp. 131-144). ACM Press/Addison-Wesley Publishing Co. doi:10.1145/344779.344849

Libelium. (2015). *50 Sensor Applications for a Smarter World.* Author.

Li, M., Yu, S., Ren, K., & Lou, W. (2010). Securing personal health records in cloud computing: Patient-centric and fine-grained data access control in multi-owner settings. In *Security and Privacy in Communication Networks* (pp. 89–106). Springer Berlin Heidelberg. doi:10.1007/978-3-642-16161-2_6

Li, M., Yu, S., Ren, K., & Lou, W. (2010). *Securing personal health records in cloud computing: Patient-centric and fine-grained data access control in multi-owner settings. In Security and Privacy in Communication Networks* (pp. 89–106). Springer.

Lin, C.-W., & Ling, Z.-H. (2007). Automatic fall incident detection in compressed video for intelligent homecare. In *Proceedings of the 16th International Conference on Computer Communications and Networks (ICCCN'07)*. doi:10.1109/ICCCN.2007.4317978

Lindemann, U., Hock, A., Stuber, M., Keck, W., & Becker, C. (2005). Evaluation of a fall detector based on accelerometers: A pilot study. *Medical & Biological Engineering & Computing, 43*(5), 548–551. doi:10.1007/BF02351026 PMID:16411625

Lin, Q., Zhang, D., Ni, H., Zhou, X., & Yu, Z. (2012). An Integrated Service Platform for Pervasive Elderly Care. In *Proceedings of the IEEE Asia-Pacific Services Computing Conference (APSCC'12)*. doi:10.1109/APSCC.2012.21

Li, Q., Stankovic, J. A., Hanson, M. A., Barth, A. T., Lach, J., & Zhou, G. (2009). Accurate, fast fall detection using gyroscopes and accelerometer-derived posture information. In *Proceedings of 6th International Workshop on Wearable and Implantable Body Sensor Networks (BSN'09)*. doi:10.1109/BSN.2009.46

Liu, C.-L., Lee, C.-H., & Lin, P.-M. (2010). A fall detection system using k-nearest neighbor classifier. *Expert Systems with Applications, 37*(10), 7174–7181. doi:10.1016/j.eswa.2010.04.014

Löhr, H., Sadeghi, A. R., & Winandy, M. (2010, November). Securing the e-health cloud. In *Proceedings of the 1st ACM International Health Informatics Symposium* (pp. 220-229). ACM.

Macmillan, R., & Dowskin, E. (2015). IBM Crafts a Role for Artificial Intelligence. *Wall Street Journal.* Retrieved January 20, 2016, from http://www.wsj.com/articles/ibm-craftsaroleforartificialintelligenceinmedicine1439265840

Macq, B., & Dewey, F. (1999, October). Trusted headers for medical images. In DFG VIII-D II Watermarking Workshop (Vol. 10). Erlangen.

Macwan, N. A., & Sajja, P. S. (2014). Fuzzy logic: An effective user interface tool for decision support system. *International Journal of Engineering Science and Innovative Technology*, *3*(3), 278–283.

Maillet, J. O., Skates, J., & Pritchett, E. (2005). American Dietetic Association: Scope of dietetics practice framework. *Journal of the American Dietetic Association*, *105*(4), 634–640. doi:10.1016/j.jada.2005.02.001 PMID:15800568

Mankad, K. B., Sajja, P. S., & Akerkar, R. A. (2011). Evolving rules using genetic fuzzy approach - An educational case study. *International Journal on Soft Computing*, *2*(1), 35–46. doi:10.5121/ijsc.2011.2104

Marks, E. (2008). *Service-Oriented Architecture (SOA) Governance for the Services Driven Enterprise*. Wiley.

Marks, E. A., & Lozano, B. (2010). *Executive's guide to cloud computing*. John Wiley and Sons.

McCann, J., Wang, H., Zheng, H., & Eccleston, C. (2012). An interactive assessment system for children with chronic pain. In *Proceedings of the IEEE-EMBS International Conference on Biomedical and Health Informatics (BHI'12)*. doi:10.1109/BHI.2012.6211739

Mccracken, G. H., Jr. (2000). Etiology and treatment of pneumonia. *Pediatric Infectious Disease Journal*, *19*(4), 373-377.

McKeown, N., Anderson, T., Balakrishnan, H., Parulkar, G., Peterson, L., Rexford, J., & Turner, J. et al. (2008). Openflow: Enabling innovation in campus networks. *SIGCOMM Comput. Commun. Rev.*, *38*(2), 69–74. doi:10.1145/1355734.1355746

Mell, P., & Grance, T. (2011). *NIST*. U.S Department of Commerce. Retrieved June 15, 2015 from http://www.nist.gov/itl/csd/cloud-102511.cfm

Mell, P., & Grance, T. (2011). *The NIST definition of cloud computing*. Retrieved from:http://csrc.nist.gov/publications/nistpubs/800-145/SP800-145.pdf

Menezes, A. J., Van Oorschot, P. C., & Vanstone, S. A. (1996). *Handbook of applied cryptography*. CRC Press. doi:10.1201/9781439821916

Microsoft. (2015). *Health vault*. Microsoft Healthvault. available: https://www.healthvault.com/in/en

Mileo, A., Merico, D., & Bisiani, R. (2010). Support for context-aware monitoring in home healthcare. *Journal of Ambient Intelligence and Smart Environments, 49-66.*

Miller, K. (2012). Big data analytics in biomedical research. *Biomedical Computation Review.*

Ming, L., Shucheng, Y., Yao, Z., Kui, R., & Wenjing, L. (2012). Scalable and Secure Sharing of Personal Health Records in Cloud Computing Using Attribute-Based Encryption. *IEEE Transactions on Parallel and Distributed Systems, 24*(1), 131–143. doi:10.1109/tpds.2012.97

Mitra, A., Rao, Y. S., & Prasanna, S. R. M. (2006). A new image encryption approach using combinational permutation techniques. *International Journal of Computer Science, 1*(2), 127–131.

Momtahan, L., Lloyd, S., & Simpson, A. (2007, June). Switched lightpaths for e-health applications: issues and challenges. In *Computer-Based Medical Systems, 2007. CBMS'07. Twentieth IEEE International Symposium on* (pp. 459-464). IEEE. doi:10.1109/CBMS.2007.104

Morrison, L. J. (1997). Major Incident Medical Management and Support: The Practical Approach. *CMAJ: Canadian Medical Association Journal, 156*(1), 78.

Msahli, M., Pujolle, G., Serhrouchni, A., Fadlallah, A., & Guenane, F. (2012, November). Openflow and on demand Networks. In *Network of the Future (NOF), 2012 Third International Conference on the* (pp. 1-5). IEEE. doi:10.1109/NOF.2012.6464006

Mu-Hsing Kuo, A. (2011). Opportunities and challenges of cloud computing to improve health care services. *Journal of Medical Internet Research.* PMID:21937354

National Institutes of Health. (n.d.). *Mediline Plus.* Retrieved February 23, 2016, from www.nlm.nih.gov/medlineplus/clinicaltrials.html

Ni, Z., Shi, Y. Q., Ansari, N., & Su, W. (2006). Reversible data hiding. *Circuits and Systems for Video Technology. IEEE Transactions on, 16*(3), 354–362.

Nutrabalance Home Page. (2014, December 19). Retrieved December 19, 2014, from Nutrabalance Web Site: http://www.nutrabalance.com/

Okuno, R., Yokoe, M., Fukawa, K., Sakoda, S., & Akazawa, K. (2007). Measurement system of finger-tapping contact force for quantitative diagnosis of Parkinson's disease. In *Proceedings of the 29th IEEE Annual International Conference of the Engineering in Medicine and Biology Society (EMBS'07).* doi:10.1109/IEMBS.2007.4352549

Ortiz, S. Jr. (2011). The problem with cloud-computing standardization. *Computer*, *44*(7), 13–16. doi:10.1109/MC.2011.220

Orwat, C., Graefe, A., & Faulwasser, T. (2008). Towards pervasive computing in health care-A literature review. *BMC Medical Informatics and Decision Making*, *8*(1), 26. doi:10.1186/1472-6947-8-26 PMID:18565221

Pal, K., Ghosh, G., & Bhattacharya, M. (2013, December). A new combined crypto-watermarking technique using RSA algorithm and discrete cosine transform to retrieve embedded EPR from noisy bio-medical images. In *Condition Assessment Techniques in Electrical Systems (CATCON), 2013 IEEE 1st International Conference on* (pp. 368-373). IEEE.

Pantelopoulos, A., & Bourbakis, N. G. (2010). A survey on wearable sensor-based systems for health monitoring and prognosis. *IEEE Transactions on Systems, Man and Cybernetics. Part C, Applications and Reviews*, *40*(1), 1–12. doi:10.1109/TSMCC.2009.2032660

Pardamean, B., & Rumanda, R. (2011). Integrated model of cloud-based e-medical record for health care organization. In *10th WSEAS International Conference on E-Activities*.

Pawar, P. S., Rajarajan, M., Nair, S. K., & Zisman, A. (2012). *Trust model for optimized cloud services* (pp. 97–112). Trust Management, VI: Springer Berlin Heidelberg.

Pérez-Freire, L., Comesana, P., & Pérez-González, F. (2005, January). Information-theoretic analysis of security in side-informed data hiding. In *Information Hiding* (pp. 131–145). Springer Berlin Heidelberg. doi:10.1007/11558859_11

Pérez-Freire, L., & Pérez-González, F. (2009). Spread-spectrum watermarking security. *Information Forensics and Security. IEEE Transactions on*, *4*(1), 2–24.

Pirahandeh, M., & Kim, D. H. (2012, April). Co-designing an intelligent doctors-colleagues-patients social network. In *Cloud Computing and Social Networking (ICCCSN), 2012 International Conference on* (pp. 1-4). IEEE. doi:10.1109/ICCCSN.2012.6215739

Poddar, R., Vishnoi, A., & Mann, V. (2015, January). HAVEN: Holistic load balancing and auto scaling in the cloud. In *Communication Systems and Networks (COMSNETS), 2015 7th International Conference on* (pp. 1-8). IEEE.

Poorejbari, S., & Vahdat-nejad, H. (2014). An Introduction to Cloud-Based Pervasive Healthcare Systems. In *4th international workshop on pervasive and context-aware middleware (PerCAM 14)*. doi:10.4108/icst.iccasa.2014.257442

Pring, B. (2011). *Forecast: Public Cloud Services, Worldwide and Regions, Industry Sectors, 2010-2015, 2011 Update.* Gartner, Inc.

Probst, Y. C., & Tapsell, L. C. (2005). Overview of computerized dietary assessment programs for research and practice in nutrition education. *Journal of Nutrition Education and Behavior*, *37*(1), 20–26. doi:10.1016/S1499-4046(06)60255-8 PMID:15745652

Pruette, C. S., Fadrowski, J. J., Bedra, M., & Finkelstein, J. (2013). Feasibility of a mobile blood pressure telemanagement system in children with hypertension. In *Proceedings of the IEEE Point-of-Care Healthcare Technologies (PHT'13)*. doi:10.1109/PHT.2013.6461316

Puech, W. (2008, October). An Efficient Hybrid Method for Safe Transfer of Medical Images. In E-MEDISYS'08: E-Medical Systems.

Puech, W., Chaumont, M., & Strauss, O. (2008, February). A reversible data hiding method for encrypted images. In *Electronic Imaging 2008* (pp. 68191E–68191E). International Society for Optics and Photonics.

Puech, W., & Rodrigues, J. M. (2004, September). A new crypto-watermarking method for medical images safe transfer. In *Signal Processing Conference, 2004 12th European* (pp. 1481-1484). IEEE.

Qian, Z., & Zhang, X. (2014). *Reversible Data Hiding in Encrypted Image with Distributed Source Encoding*. Academic Press.

Rakocevic, G. (2009). Overview of sensors for wireless sensor networks. *Transactions on Internet Research*, *5*, 13–18.

Ran, L., Helal, S., & Moore, S. (2004). Drishti: an integrated indoor/outdoor blind navigation system and service. In *Proceedings of the 2nd IEEE Annual Conference on Pervasive Computing and Communications (PerCom'04)* doi:10.1109/PERCOM.2004.1276842

Rantz, M., Skubic, M., Koopman, R., Phillips, L., Alexander, G., Miller, S., & Guevara, R. (2011). Using sensor networks to detect urinary tract infections in older adults. In *13th International Conference on e-Health Networking, Application and Services*. doi:10.1109/HEALTH.2011.6026731

Rao, N. V., & Kumari, V. M. (2011). Watermarking in medical imaging for security and authentication. *Information Security Journal: A Global Perspective, 20*(3), 148-155.

Rashidi, P., & Mihailidis, A. (2013). A survey on ambient-assisted living tools for older adults. *IEEE Journal of Biomedical and Health Informatics, 17*(3), 579-590.

Rashidi, P., & Cook, D. J. (2009). Keeping the Resident in the Loop: Adapting the Smart Home to the User. *IEEE Transactions on Systems, Man, and Cybernetics. Part A, Systems and Humans, 39*(5), 949–959. doi:10.1109/TSMCA.2009.2025137

Ratnam, K. A., & Dominic, P. D. D. (2012). Cloud services - Enhancing the Malaysian healthcare sector. In *Proceedings of the International Conference on Computer & Information Science (ICCIS'12)*.

Recommendation, X. (2000). *509-The Directory: Public-key and attribute certificate frameworks*. International Telecommunication Union.

Rimminen, H., Lindström, J., Linnavuo, M., & Sepponen, R. (2010). Detection of falls among the elderly by a floor sensor using the electric near field. *IEEE Transactions on Information Technology in Biomedicine, 14*(6), 1475-1476.

Rittinghouse, J., & Ransome, J. (2009). *Cloud Computing: Implementation, Management, and Security*. CRC Press, Inc.

Rolim, C. O., Koch, F. L., Westphall, C. B., Werner, J., Fracalossi, A., & Salvador, G. S. (2010). A Cloud Computing Solution for Patient's Data Collection in Health Care Institutions. In *Proceedings of the Second International Conference on eHealth, Telemedicine, and Social Medicine* (ETELEMED '10).

Sadeghi, A. R. (2008). The marriage of cryptography and watermarking—beneficial and challenging for secure watermarking and detection. In *Digital Watermarking* (pp. 2–18). Springer Berlin Heidelberg. doi:10.1007/978-3-540-92238-4_2

Sajja, P. S. (2011). Personalized content representation through hybridization of mobile agent and interface agent. In S. Bagchi & S. Bagchi (Eds.), *Ubiquitous Multimedia and Mobile Agents: Models and Implementations* (pp. 85–112). Hershey, PA: IGI Global Book Publishing.

Sajja, P. S., & Akerkar, R. (2013). Bio-inspired models and the semantic web. In Z. C. Xin-She Yang & Z. C. Xin-She Yang (Eds.), *Swarm Intelligence and Bio-Inspired Computation: Theory and Applications* (pp. 273–294). Waltham, MA: Elsevier. doi:10.1016/B978-0-12-405163-8.00012-0

Sajja, P. S., & Trivedi, J. (2010). Using type-2 hyperbolic tangent activation function in artificial neural network. *Research Lines, 3*(2), 51–57.

Saldarriaga, A. J., Pérez, J. J., Restrepo, J., & Bustamante, J. (2013, April). A mobile application for ambulatory electrocardiographic monitoring in clinical and domestic environments. In Health Care Exchanges (PAHCE), 2013 Pan American (pp. 1-4). IEEE. doi:10.1109/PAHCE.2013.6568306

Salsano, S., Ventre, P. L., Prete, L., Siracusano, G., Gerola, M., & Salvadori, E. (2014, September). OSHI-Open Source Hybrid IP/SDN networking (and its emulation on Mininet and on distributed SDN testbeds). In *Software Defined Networks (EWSDN), 2014 Third European Workshop on* (pp. 13-18). IEEE.

Sandström, B. (2001). A framework for food-based dietary guidelines in the European Union. *Public Health Nutrition, 4*(2A), 293–305. PMID:11688435

Schneier, B. (2007). *Applied cryptography: protocols, algorithms, and source code in C*. John Wiley & Sons.

Schneier, B. (1996). *Applied cryptography*. New York: Wiley.

Schultz, T. (2013). Turning healthcare challenges into big data opportunities: A use-case review across the pharmaceutical development lifecycle. *Bull. Association Inform. Sci. Technol., 39*, 34–40. doi:10.1002/bult.2013.1720390508

Sen, R. (2015). Building smarter wearable's for health-care. *IBM Developer Works*. Retrieved January 15, 2016, from http://www.ibm.com/developerworks/library/cc-smarter-wearables-healthcare-concepts/index.html

Shadab Ansari, W., Alamri, A. M., Hassan, M., & Shoaib, M. (2013). A survey on sensor-cloud: Architecture, Applications and Approaches. *International Journal of Distributed Sensor Networks*.

Shahid, Z., Chaumont, M., & Puech, W. (2011). Fast protection of H. 264/AVC by selective encryption of CAVLC and CABAC for I and P frames. *Circuits and Systems for Video Technology. IEEE Transactions on, 21*(5), 565–576.

Shaou-Gang, M., Pei-Hsu, S., & Chia-Yuan, H. (2006). A Customized Human Fall Detection System Using Omni-Camera Images and Personal Information. In *Proceedings of the 1st Transdisciplinary Conference on Distributed Diagnosis and Home Healthcare* (D2H2'06).

Shima, K., Tamura, Y., Tsuji, T., Kandori, A., Yokoe, M., & Sakoda, S. (2008). Estimation of human finger tapping forces based on a fingerpad-stiffness model. In *Proceedings of the IEEE Annual International Conference of the Engineering in Medicine and Biology Society (EMBC'09)*.

Shima, K., Tsuji, T., Kandori, A., Yokoe, M., & Sakoda, S. (2009). Measurement and evaluation of finger tapping movements using log-linearized Gaussian mixture networks. *Sensors (Basel, Switzerland)*, *9*(3), 2187–2201. doi:10.3390/s90302187 PMID:22574008

Shimrat, O. (2009). Cloud computing and healthcare. *San Diego Physician. Org*, 26-29.

Shucheng, Y., Cong, W., Kui, R., & Wenjing, L. (2010). Achieving Secure, Scalable, and Fine-grained Data Access Control in Cloud Computing. In *Proceedings of the IEEE INFOCOM*.

Singh, S., Puradkar, S., & Lee, Y. (2006). Ubiquitous Computing: Connecting Pervasive Computing through Semantic web. *Information Systems and e-Business Management, 4*(4), 421-439.

Singh, H., Naik, A. D., Rao, R., & Petersen, L. A. (2008). Reducing diagnostic errors through effective communication: Harnessing the power of information technology. *Journal of General Internal Medicine*, *23*(4), 489–494. doi:10.1007/s11606-007-0393-z PMID:18373151

Starida, K., Ganiatsas, G., Fotiadis, D. I., & Likas, A. (2003). CHILDCARE: a collaborative environment for the monitoring of children healthcare at home. In *Proceedings of the 4th International IEEE EMBS Special Topic Conference on Information Technology Applications in Biomedicine*. doi:10.1109/ITAB.2003.1222501

Stein, K. (2010). Nutrition beyond the numbers: Counseling clients on nutrient value interpretation. *Journal of the Academy of Nutrition and Dietetics*, *110*(12), 1800–1803. PMID:21111084

Stinson, D. R. (2005). *Cryptography: theory and practice*. CRC Press.

Struijk, L. N. S. A. (2006). An inductive tongue computer interface for control of computers and assistive devices. *IEEE Transactions on Bio-Medical Engineering*, *53*(12), 2594–2597. doi:10.1109/TBME.2006.880871 PMID:17152438

Sultan, N. (2013). Making use of cloud computing for healthcare provision: Opportunities and challenges. *International Journal of Information Management, 34*(2), 177–184. doi:10.1016/j.ijinfomgt.2013.12.011

Super, G., Groth, S., & Hook, R. (1994). *START: simple triage and rapid treatment plan*. Newport Beach, CA: Hoag Memorial Presbyterian Hospital.

Takami, O., Morimoto, K., Ochiai, T., & Ishimatsu, T. (1995). Computer interface to use head and eyeball movement for handicapped people. In *Proceedings of the IEEE International Conference on Intelligent Systems for the 21st Century, Systems, Man and Cybernetics*. doi:10.1109/ICSMC.1995.537920

Takami, O., Irie, N., Kang, C., Ishimatsu, T., & Ochiai, T. (1996). Computer interface to use head movement for handicapped people. In *Proceedings of the IEEE TENCON on Digital Signal Processing Applications (TENCON'96)*. doi:10.1109/ TENCON.1996.608861

Tamura, T., Kawarada, A., Nambu, M., Tsukada, A., Sasaki, K., & Yamakoshi, K. I. (2007). E-healthcare at an experimental welfare techno house in Japan. *Open Medical Informatics*, 1-7.

Tartamella, S. S., Pruehsner, W., & Enderle, J. D. (1999). Remote control digital thermostat and remote door opener. In *Proceedings of the IEEE 25th Annual Northeast Bioengineering Conference*. doi:10.1109/NEBC.1999.755759

Terry, N. P. (2013). Protecting patient privacy in the age of big data. *UMKC Law Review, 81*, 385–415.

Thodi, D. M., & Rodriguez, J. J. (2004, October). Prediction-error based reversible watermarking. In *Image Processing, 2004. ICIP'04. 2004 International Conference on* (Vol. 3, pp. 1549-1552). IEEE. doi:10.1109/ICIP.2004.1421361

Tian, J. (2003). Reversible data embedding using a difference expansion. *IEEE Transactions on Circuits and Systems for Video Technology, 13*(8), 890–896. doi:10.1109/TCSVT.2003.815962

Toosi, A. N., Calheiros, R. N., & Buyya, R. (2014). *Interconnected cloud computing environments: Challenges, taxonomy, and survey. In ACM Computing Surveys*. CSUR.

Tourrilhes, J., Sharma, P., Banerjee, S., & Pettit, J. (2014). SDN and OpenFlow Evolution: A Standards Perspective. *Computer, 47*(11), 22–29. doi:10.1109/MC.2014.326

Trivedi, J. A., & Sajja, P. S. (2011). Improving efficiency of round robin scheduling using neuro fuzzy approach. *International Journal of Research and Reviews in Computer Science, 2*(2), 308–311.

Trivedi, J. A., & Sajja, P. S. (2011). Online guidance for effective investment using type-2 fuzzy neuro advisory system. *International Journal of Computer Science and Information Technologies, 2*(2), 799–803.

UNICEF. (2008). *Countdown to 2015. Tracking progress in maternal, neonatal and child survival: the 2008 report*. New York: UNICEF.

Uniyal, D., & Raychoudhury, V. (2014). *Pervasive Healthcare-A Comprehensive Survey of Tools and Techniques*. arXiv preprint arXiv:1411.1821

US Department of Health and Human Services. (2008). *The ONC-Coordinated Federal Health IT Strategic Plan: 2008-2012*. US Department of Health and Human Services.

Vahdat-nejad, H., Zamanifar, K., & Nematbakhsh, N. (2013). Context-aware middleware architecture for smart home environment. *International Journal of Smart Home, 7*, 77-86.

Vaquero, L., Rodero-Merino, L., Caceres, J., & Lindner, M. (2008). A break in the clouds: Towards a cloud definition. *SIGCOMM Comput. Commun. Rev., 39*(1), 50–55. doi:10.1145/1496091.1496100

Varshney, U. (2007). Pervasive healthcare and wireless health monitoring. *Mobile Networks and Applications, 12*(2-3), 113–127. doi:10.1007/s11036-007-0017-1

Varshney, U. (2009). *Pervasive Healthcare Computing: EMR/EHR*. Wireless and Health Monitoring. doi:10.1007/978-1-4419-0215-3

Velte, A., Velte, T., & Elsenpeter, R. (2010). *Cloud Computing A Practical Approach*. McGraw-Hill.

Vishwakarma, V., Mandal, C., & Sural, S. (2007). *Automatic detection of human fall in video. In Pattern Recognition and Machine Intelligence* (pp. 616–623). Springer. doi:10.1007/978-3-540-77046-6_76

Visintin, M., Barbeau, H., Korner-Bitensky, N., & Mayo, N. E. (1998). A new approach to retrain gait in stroke patients through body weight support and treadmill stimulation. *Stroke, 29*(6), 1122–1128. doi:10.1161/01.STR.29.6.1122 PMID:9626282

Wang, S. Y. (2014, June). Comparison of SDN OpenFlow network simulator and emulators: EstiNet vs. Mininet. In *Computers and Communication (ISCC), 2014 IEEE Symposium on* (pp. 1-6). IEEE.

Wan, J., Zou, C., Ullah, S., Lai, C., Zhou, M., & Wang, X. (2013). Cloud-Enabled wireless body area networks for pervasive healthcare. *IEEE Network*, 27(5), 56–61. doi:10.1109/MNET.2013.6616116

Warner, D. (2013). *Safe de-identification of big data is critical to health care.* Health Inform. Manage.

White, S.E., (2014). A review of big data in health care: Challenges and opportunities. *Open Access Bio inform., 6*, 13-18. DOI: 10.2147/OAB.S50519

WHO. (2007). *Global report on falls prevention in older age.* World Health Organization.

WHO. (2015a). *The 10 leading causes of death in the world, 2000 and 2012.* Retrieved from http://www.who.int/mediacentre/factsheets/fs310/en/

WHO. (2015b). World Health Organization.

William, S., & Stallings, W. (2006). *Cryptography and Network Security, 4/E.* Pearson Education India.

Williams, A., Ganesan, D., & Hanson, A. (2007). Aging in place: fall detection and localization in a distributed smart camera network. In *Proceedings of the 15th International Conference on Multimedia.* doi:10.1145/1291233.1291435

Wood, A., Stankovic, J. A., Virone, G., Selavo, L., He, Z., Cao, Q., & Stoleru, R. et al. (2008). Context-aware wireless sensor networks for assisted living and residential monitoring. *IEEE Network, 22*(4), 26–33. doi:10.1109/MNET.2008.4579768

Woon Ahn, Y., Cheng, A. M. K., Baek, J., Jo, M., & Chen, H. (2013). An auto-scaling mechanism for virtual resources to support mobile, pervasive, real-time healthcare applications in cloud computing. *IEEE Network, 27*(5), 62–68. doi:10.1109/MNET.2013.6616117

World Health Organization. (2012). *International classification of diseases.* ICD.

Wu, H. T., & Cheung, Y. M. (2005, September). A reversible data hiding approach to mesh authentication. In *Web Intelligence, 2005. Proceedings. The 2005 IEEE/WIC/ACM International Conference on* (pp. 774-777). IEEE.

Wu, H. T., & Cheung, Y. M. (2010). Reversible watermarking by modulation and security enhancement. *Instrumentation and Measurement. IEEE Transactions on*, *59*(1), 221–228.

Xuan, G., Zhu, J., Chen, J., Shi, Y. Q., Ni, Z., & Su, W. (2002). Distortionless data hiding based on integer wavelet transform. *Electronics Letters*, *38*(25), 1646–1648. doi:10.1049/el:20021131

Yang, S., Njoku, M., & Mackenzie, C. F. (2014). 'Big data' approaches to trauma outcome prediction and autonomous resuscitation. *British Journal of Hospital Medicine*, *75*(11), 637–641. doi:10.12968/hmed.2014.75.11.637 PMID:25383434

Yoo, E.-H., & Lee, S.-Y. (2010). Glucose biosensors: An overview of use in clinical practice. *Sensors (Basel, Switzerland)*, *10*, 4558–4576. doi:10.3390/s100504558

Yu, S., Wang, C., Ren, K., & Lou, W. (2010, March). Achieving secure, scalable, and fine-grained data access control in cloud computing. In Infocom, 2010 proceedings IEEE (pp. 1-9). IEEE. doi:10.1109/INFCOM.2010.5462174

Yu, K.-H., Yoon, M.-J., & Jeong, G.-Y. (2013). Recognition of obstacle distribution via vibrotactile stimulation for the visually disabled. In *Proceedings of the IEEE International Conference on Mechatronics (ICM'13)*

Zadeh, L. A. (1965). Fuzzy sets. *Information and Control*, *8*(3), 338–353. doi:10.1016/S0019-9958(65)90241-X

Zeghid, M., Machhout, M., Khriji, L., Baganne, A., & Tourki, R. (2007). A modified AES based algorithm for image encryption. *International Journal on Computer Science and Engineering*, *1*(1), 70–75.

Zhang, C., Tian, Y., & Capezuti, E. (2012). *Privacy preserving automatic fall detection for elderly using RGBD cameras*. Springer. doi:10.1007/978-3-642-31522-0_95

Zhang, G., & Liu, Q. (2011). A novel image encryption method based on total shuffling scheme. *Optics Communications*, *284*(12), 2775–2780. doi:10.1016/j.optcom.2011.02.039

Zhang, R., Lee, M., & Liu, L. (2010). Security models and requirements for healthcare application clouds. In *3rd International Conference on Cloud Computing*. doi:10.1109/CLOUD.2010.62

Zhang, W., Ma, K., & Yu, N. (2014). Reversibility improved data hiding in encrypted images. *Signal Processing*, *94*, 118–127. doi:10.1016/j.sigpro.2013.06.023

Zhang, X. (2011). Reversible data hiding in encrypted image. *Signal Processing Letters, IEEE*, *18*(4), 255–258. doi:10.1109/LSP.2011.2114651

Zhang, Y., Lee, M., & Gatton, T. M. (2009). Agent-Based Healthcare Systems for Real-Time Chronic Diseases. In *2009 World Conference on Services-I*. doi:10.1109/SERVICES-I.2009.104

Zhu, Z. L., Zhang, W., Wong, K. W., & Yu, H. (2011). A chaos-based symmetric image encryption scheme using a bit-level permutation. *Information Sciences*, *181*(6), 1171–1186. doi:10.1016/j.ins.2010.11.009

Ziefle, M., & Rocker, C. (2010). Acceptance of pervasive healthcare systems: A Comparison of Different Implementation Concepts. In *4th international conference on pervasive computing*. doi:10.4108/ICST.PERVASIVEHEALTH2010.8915

About the Contributors

Chintan M. Bhatt is currently working as an Assistant Professor in Computer Engineering Department, Chandubhai S. Patel Institute of Technology, CHARUSAT. He is a member of IEEE, EAI, ACM, CSI, AIRCC (Academy & Industry Research Collaboration Center) and IAENG (International Association of Engineers). His areas of interest include Internet of Things, Data Mining, Web Mining, Networking, Security Mobile Computing, Big Data and Software Engineering. He has more than 5 years of teaching experience and research experience, having good teaching and research interests. He has chaired a track in CSNT 2015 and ICTCS 2014. He has been working as Reviewer in Wireless Communications, IEEE (Impact Factor-6.524) and Internet of Things Journal, IEEE, Knowledge-Based Systems, Elsevier (Impact Factor-2.9) Applied Computing and Informatics, Elsevier and Mobile Networks and Applications, Springer. He has delivered an expert talk on "Internet of Things" at Broadcast Engineering Society Doordarshan, Ahmedabad on 30/09/2015. He has been awarded Faculty with Maximum Publication in CSIC Award and Paper Presenter Award at International Conference in CSI-2015, held at New Delhi.

Sateesh K. Peddoju has an overall professional experience of nearly 18 years and working currently with Department of Computer Science and Engineering, Indian Institute of Technology Roorkee, Roorkee, India. His areas of research include Cloud Computing, Mobile Computing and their Security Issues. He obtained his Master's and Doctoral degrees from Osmania University, Hyderabad. He is contributing to the society through various International/National Technical societies such as ACM, IEEE, IEEE CS, DMTF and CSI. He is acting as Vice-Chair for IEEE Computer Society, India Council and Faculty Sponsor for ACM IITR Students Chapter. He is also the Faculty Advisor for Software Development Section of Hobbies Club at IIT Roorkee. IBM has honored him with Shared University Research Award for the year 2013. He is also honored with Best Teacher Award when he was working with a private engineering college. He secured University 4th rank in his Master's degree. His research contribution is demonstrated by his various publications (over 50) through standard publishers like ACM/IEEE/Springer/Elsevier, some received awards, including peer-reviewed journals and conferences. He is executing sponsored projects of total worth around 50 lakhs. He is the editorial board member for several journals and reviewer for popular journals from Elsevier, Springer, Inderscience and IGI Global. He is also editing a book on "Cloud Computing Systems and Applications in Healthcare" to be published by IGI Global. He has wide experience inConference/Workshop management at the capacity of General Chair/Program Chair/Session Chair/TPC/Keynote Speaker. He has been the expert committee member at national level including DOEACC (now, NIELIT) and for several universities like Uttarakhand Technical University and Mahamaya Technical University. He is also Board of Studies member for "Electronics and Computers" courses for Jawaharlal Technological University, Anantapur. So far, he has supervised 30+ M.Tech projects, 35+ B.Tech projects. Currently, he is supervising 9 Ph.D students out of which 2 students have already submitted the thesis. He has visited several countries like United States, United Kingdom, and South Korea. He has very high network of collaborations throughout the world across several universities. He has been teaching several courses like Cloud Computing, Mobile and Pervasive Computing, Advanced Computer Networks, Network Security, and Operating Systems at UG and PG level students.

* * *

Mayank Aggarwal is presently working as Assistant Professor/Incharge Computer Sc. & Engineering at Faculty of Engineering & Technology, Gurukul Kangri University, Haridwar. He was designated as IBM Cloud Consultant for 2015 by Channel Technologies. Has an experience of 13 years in academics. He is IBM Bluemix (IBM Cloud) certified and Microsoft Azure Certified by MaGe. He was awarded by IBM TGMC mentor Award-2013. He has represented Uttarakhand, U.P. West and Himachal as Science Communicator in Indian Science Congress-2014. He has been a gold medalist and university topper in B.Tech after that he got his M.Tech and Ph.D. degree. He has more than 20 papers to his credit in reputed journals / Conferences. He has been Organizing Secretary and Co-Organizing Secretary for many conferences/international conferences. He has conducted several workshops in the field of Cloud Computing and "How to make Science Accessible to Common Man" in various colleges/ universities. He is a resource person in Academic

Staff College, Kumaon University, Nainital. He has been awarded "Best Teacher of Computer Sc. & Engineering Award – 2014" and also "Most Popular Teacher of Faculty of Engineering &Technology Award" for 2011,2104. He is a Life Member of CSI, IETE, ISCA.He is also involved in various social activities and is an active member of Red Cross and Bharat Vikas Parishad.

Nagaraju Aitha received a M.Sc(Pure Maths) from the Central University of Hyderabad in 1998; M.Tech in Computer Science and Technology from University of Mysore, and Ph.D From Osmania University, Hyderabad. His research area includes Software Defined Networks(SDN) and Cloud Computing. He has published 25 conference papers 10 peer reviewed journals. He worked as various positions from 2002-12 in two engineering colleges affiliated to JNTU, Hyderabad. At present He is working as Assistant Professor in Computer Science at Central University of Rajasthan since 2012. The University appointed as NKN Coordinator to perform the objectives of NKN. He has established a Remote Center to conduct online workshops using blended mode which is T10kT Project initiated by MHRD-IITB. He is School Board member for two Schools in Central University of Rajasthan.

Anna Babu was born in Ernakulam, Kerala, India, in 1989. She received her Bachelor's degree in Computer Science and Engineering from University of Calicut of Kerala, India, in 2010. She also received her Master's in Information Systems from M. G. University, Kerala, India in 2015. From 2010 to 2012 she had worked with mobile industry as Mobile Application Developer after which she enrolled for her Master's in 2013. Since 2015 she has been an Assistant Professor in college affiliated to M.G. University, Kerala, India. Her areas of research include Crypto-Watermarking techniques, Security in Health Care and Cyber Security.

Balamurugan Balusamy completed his B.E(computer science and Engineering) from Bharathidasan University and M.E(Computer Science) from Anna University. He did his Ph.D. in computer science in the area of cloud access control from VIT University. His research interests are Cloud Computing,IOT and Big data and strives hard to connect all of them together.

Ajay Chaudhary has an overall professional teaching and research experience of more than 10 years and currently working as Assistant Professor in Department of IT, Govt. Engineering College, Bikaner. He obtained his graduate degree from University of Rajasthan, Jaipur in 2005 and Master's in Computer Science & Engineering from IIT(Indian Institute of Technology), Roorkee in 2011. He currently is pursuing Doctoral degree from Indian Institute of Technology, Roorkee. His area of research includes Cloud Computing, Wireless Sensor Networks, Internet of Things (IoT), Computer Networking, Security, Intrusion detection & Prevention systems(IDS & IPS). He is a member of various International/National Technical societies such as ACM, ACM CSTA, IACSIT, IAENG, ISTE and IGC. He has visited several countries like South Korea and Hong Kong. He participated in more than 50 courses, workshops, symposiums and conferences etc. He has conducted several one and two-week short term courses and workshops. He publishes several papers in reputed peer-reviewed conferences and journals of standard publishers like ACM/IEEE/Springer. He acts as Technical program committee and organizing committee member of several reputable conferences of ACM/Springer. He has reviewed various international reputed journals papers and conferences and book chapters.

Drashti Dave received her BTech degree in Information Technology from University of Rajasthan, in 2006, and the MTech degree in Computer Science & Engineering from Pacific University in 2012. From 2007 to 2008, she has worked as Network Administrator in Rainbow Telecom (now MTS) From 2008 to 2014, she worked as a Faculty in the Department of Computer Science & Engineering, College of Technology and Engineering. At present she is pursuing PhD degree from the Central University of Rajasthan. She has published 2 International Conference paper. Her research interests include Software Defined Network, Information Security and Network Security.

Charu Gandhi is an associate professor at the Department of Computer Science and Information Technology, Jaypee Institute of Information Technology, JIIT Noida India. She received a PhD degree in Computer Science & Engineering from Kurukshetra University, Haryana, India, M.Tech degree in Computer Science from Banasthali Vidyapith, Rajasthan, India and a B.Tech degree in Computer Science & Engineering from from Kurukshetra University, Haryana, India. Her research interests include wireless and sensor network, mobile network, network security and cloud computing. She also participated in many international Conferences. She has published several papers in national and international conferences and journals. She has authored or co-authored over 10 papers in international journals.

Shweta Kaushik is an assistant professor at the Department of Computer Science and Technology, IP University of Delhi. She pursuing her PhD degree in Computer Science & Engineering from, Jaypee Institute of Information Technology, JIIT Noide India. She received a M.Tech degree in Computer Science from JIIT Noida, Uttar

Pradesh, India and a B.Tech degree in Computer Science & Engineering from Uttar Pradesh Technical University, Uttar Pradesh, India. Her research interests include network security, Distributed System, Algorithms, Big data and cloud computing. She also participated in many international Conferences. She has published several papers in national and international conferences and journals. She has authored or co-authored for many papers in international journals. She is also an active member of ACM.

Mani Madhukar is Cloud Partner Leader at IBM India Pvt. Ltd. His work area relates to development of Ecosystem for adoption of IBM Cloud platform. He is a regular speaker and evangelist at various national and international platforms on areas including Cloud computing, Big Data, Internet of Things, Cognitive computing and Watson Analytics. He is a member of numerous committees and boards in various universities representing IBM and assisting academic establishments in incorporating latest trends in technology in academic learning. He has experience in the domains of Cloud, ECM, IDP and IOT. His current research interests include cognitive computing, social media analytics and recommender systems.

Wathiq Mansoor is a Professor of computer engineering and the director of education and research for smart technologies CREST at the American University in Dubai. He earned his Ph.D. in computer science and engineering from Aston University in UK. His doctoral work was on the design and implementations of multiprocessors systems for computer vision. His master and master thesis is the treatment of Epilepsy using Bio-feedback. He has published many research papers in the area of biomedical engineering, context aware systems, ubiquitous computing, web services, neural networks, and computer networks. He has organized tens of international conferences and workshops.

Sepideh Poorejbari is a researcher at Pervasive & Cloud Computing research Lab at the University of Birjand (PerLab). She received her master degree from computer engineering department of Islamic Azad University of Birjand, Iran, in 2015, her bachelor's degree from Sadjad University of Technology, Mashhad, Iran, in 2007. Currently, her research is focused on distributed systems and cloud computing specially in healthcare sector. She has published a survey paper in "4th International Workshop on Pervasive and Context-aware middleware" (2014, Dubai) and participated in different conferences and workshops.

Priti Srinivas Sajja (b.1970) joined the faculty of the Department of Computer Science, Sardar Patel University, India in 1994 and presently working as a Professor. She received her M.S. (1993) and Ph.D (2000) in Computer Science from the Sardar Patel University. Her research interests include knowledge-based systems, soft computing, multiagent systems, and software engineering. She has 169 publications in books, book chapters, journals, and in the proceedings of national and international conferences out of which five publications have won best research paper awards. She is co-author of 'Knowledge-Based Systems' and 'Intelligent Technologies for Web Applications' published at USA. She is supervising work of a few doctoral research scholars while six candidates have completed their Ph.D research under her guidance. She was Principal Investigator of a major research project funded by UGC, India. She is serving as a member in editorial board of many international science journals and served as program committee member for various international conferences.

S. C. Sharma received M.Sc. (Electronics), M. Tech. (Electronics & Communication Engg.) and Ph.D. (Electronics & Computer Engg.) in 1981, 1983 and 1992 respectively from IIT Roorkee (erstwhile University of Roorkee). He started his career as R & D Engineer in 1983 then joined teaching profession in Jan. 1984 at IIT-Roorkee and continuing till date. He has published over two hundred twenty research papers in national and international journals(107)/conferences(115) and supervised more than 30 projects/dissertation of PG students. He has supervised 14 Ph.D. in the area of Computer Networking, Wireless Network, Computer Communication and continuing supervising Ph.D. in the same area. He has successfully completed several major research projects independently funded by various Govt. Agencies like AICTE, CSIR, UGC, MHRD, DST, DRDO, UKCOST and many minor research projects related to Communication and SAW filter design sponsored by the Government of India. IIT-Roorkee has awarded him the Khosla annual research prize with the best research paper. His many research papers have been awarded by National and International Committees and Journals. Recently one of the thesis of his student has been awarded the best thesis of the year-2012 by springer. He has worked as a research scientist at FMH, Munchen, Germany and visited many countries (UK, France, Germany, Italy, Switzerland, Canada, UAE, Thailand etc) related to research work. He has chaired session of International Conferences and deliverd invited talk at various forums. He is the active reviewer of the IEEE Sensor Journal and Chief Editor of various reputed International Journals and Editor of many

National Journal. He is the honorary member of IEEE, NSBE, ISOC and IAENG, USA. He has also worked as group leader (Head) of Electronics & Instrumentation Engg. Department of BITS-Pilani-Dubai Campus, from Aug. 2003 to Aug. 2005. Presently he is continuing as Professor at IIT Roorkee.

Jeegar Ashokkumar Trivedi obtained his doctorate degree in the field of Computer Science from Sardar Patel University, Gujarat, India. He specializes in Artificial Intelligence especially in Neuro-Fuzzy Systems. He has also developed a framework to develop Neuro-Fuzzy System in specified domain area as a part of his research work. He has published more than 15 International and National journal papers. He is an active researcher and presently rendering his services to Post Graduate Department of Computer Science & Technology, Sardar Patel University, Gujarat, India.

Hamed Vahdat-Nejad is currently an assistant professor at the computer engineering department of the University of Birjand. He received his PhD from computer engineering department of University of Isfahan in 2012, his master degree from Ferdowsi University of Mashhad in 2007, and his bachelor's degree from Sharif University of Technology in 2004. He was a research scholar at the Middleware laboratory of Sapienza University of Rome in 2011. Currently, his research is focused on context-awareness as well as related domains such as healthcare. He has (co)published about30 papers in conferences and journals, and leads the Pervasive & Cloud computing research Lab at the University of Birjand. He has served as the chairman of the 1st & 2nd International Workshop on Context-aware Middleware for Ubiquitous Computing Environments, as well as the "3rd & 4th International workshop on Pervasive and Context-aware middleware". He has served as TPC member for ICCKE, IWCMC, ISIEA, ICCIT-WCS, PerCAM, ChinaCOM, MELECON2014, COGNITIVE-2014,IBMSGS2015, EMERGING 2015,ICACCI,ADMMET'2015 ICCME-2015, CoCoNet'15, AR4MET'2016, REEGETECH'2016, ISTA'16, etc. Currently, he serves as guest editor for Elsevier Computers and electrical engineering journal and Journal of Computing and Security.

Rajya Lakshmi Gubburi Venkataramana, received the Master of Science in Software Engineering at the Vellore Institute of Technology, India in 2014 and her Second Master's in Computer Science at the Northwestern Polytechnic University, United States in 2016 specialization in Cloud computing. She also received Achiever Award for Excellence in student academic and as a young researcher from Dr. Vishwanathan Honor Chancellor of VIT University, India. She recently received Upsilon Pi Epsilon (UPE) Excellence Award in recognition of exemplary involvement in excellent research achievement, and participation in extracurricular activities relevant to the computing discipline from IEEE Computer Society. Additionally, she published 13 papers in very competitive conferences and journals in the filed of cloud computing and computer science applications. Ms. Rajya is an enthusiastic young researcher to find an innovative solution in cloud data Optimization.

Index

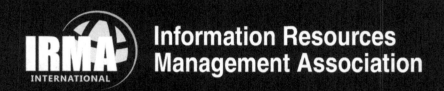
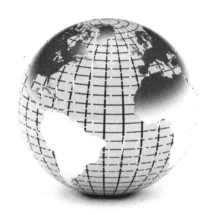

Printed in the United States
By Bookmasters